FOOD FOR SPORT

FOOD FOR SPORT
EAT WELL, PERFORM BETTER

Jane Griffin

The Crowood Press

First published in 2001 by
The Crowood Press Ltd
Ramsbury, Marlborough
Wiltshire SN8 2HR

www.crowood.com

This impression 2004

British Library Cataloguing-in-Publication Data
A catalogue record for this book is available from the British Library.

ISBN 1 86126 216 7

Line drawings by Annette Findlay

Photographs © EMPICS

Note
Whilst every effort has been made to ensure that this book is
technically accurate and sound, neither the author nor the publisher
can accept responsibility for any injury or loss sustained as a result of
using this material.

Typeset by Phoenix Typesetting, Burley-in-Wharfedale, West Yorkshire.

Printed and bound in Great Britain by J. W. Arrowsmith Ltd.

Contents

Foreword

I have been involved with elite sport, in particular rowing, for the past fifteen years, initially as a competitor, then as a medic. Increasingly I have become aware of the relevance of good diet to realising sporting potential at whatever level you are aiming. A good diet enables you to train well, perform well and stay healthy. It allows the immune system to protect you and enhances recovery from illness or injury. In sports where 'making weight' is necessary, an understanding of the components of a good diet and the interaction between these components allows weight to be lost effectively whilst maintaining performance.

Accessing good dietetic information is not always easy. I welcome this book as an innovation for anybody involved in sport.

Eat well, perform well.

Dr Lady Redgrave
Chief Medical Officer,
Great Britain Rowing Team

Acknowledgements

To my husband Chris for his love, patience and support.

To my children Daniel and Jessica for their love and encouragement.

To Vivian Grisogono and Craig Sharp for putting me on the sports nutrition road all those years ago.

To my friends at Ealing Squash Club for knowing when to stop asking if the book was finished.

And last but by no means least to all the sportsmen and -women I have worked with. This book is born out of what I have learnt from working with them. It is dedicated to them.

Introduction

Regular physical activity is good for us, and so is food. Apart from many major health benefits, being more physically active can make food more enjoyable. The more active you are, the more energy you use, so the more food you need and can eat without gaining excess weight. Given that the incidence of overweight and obesity is steadily rising and yet we are on average eating less, the role of physical activity and a supporting healthy diet becomes very apparent.

Many people maintain their physical activity level through a pursuit of a sport, or several sports. For the majority, this is enjoyed at a recreational or club level but for a few, sport is their livelihood. Some dream of representing their country or competing at a World Championships or Olympic Games, although only a very small number make it. We all have our goals, perhaps to win the tennis club mixed doubles final or to run a personal best (PB) half marathon time, or perhaps just to be playing as much squash in ten years' time as we do today.

Regardless of the level at which you participate or compete, diet can play an enormous part in improving performance. What, when and how much you eat and drink can have a direct effect on your sporting performance.

- If you don't get your diet right, you could run out of energy before the end of a training session, match, race or competition. If you are tired you won't put in your best performance, both physically and mentally.
- If you don't get your diet right, you could be putting yourself at greater risk of getting injured during a training session or competition.
- In a competition, getting your diet right could give you the edge over your opposition. In the closing minutes you want to be the one edging ahead, not your opponent.
- Getting your diet right can also help in recovery from injury and illness.
- By coincidence, the basis of the diet that is best for sporting performance bears many similarities with the general advice for long-term health. This may not be your major concern at the moment, but at least you can be reassured that you are doing yourself a health favour as well as benefiting your performance.

This book is designed so that you can pick up at whatever point suits you. Chapters 1 to 3 discuss basic nutrition and physiology as a foundation for the following chapters. Throughout the book, nutrition is treated in relation to food so that you can build up the appropriate diet for your own needs. You will learn not only how to eat for your sport but why you should eat in this way. If you understand the theory behind the practical advice, you are much more likely to follow the advice.

Chapters 4 to 7 build on the basics, linking into the physiology to show how the training and competition diet can help prevent fatigue, help recovery and prevent injury. Changes to body weight and body fat can improve performance, although some diets take weight loss to unnecessary and unhealthy extremes. Weight or body fat loss can be achieved without a loss of sporting performance but not all the diets promoted to the general public are appropriate to sportspersons, as you will see. The dietary supplement and ergogenic (performance enhancing) aids market is investigated but, as new products are constantly being launched, this section also gives guidance on how to evaluate such products for yourself.

In Chapters 8 to 13 the potential problems that can be associated with certain population groups or situations are highlighted and practical ways in which these problems can be resolved by diet are shown. The information given in these chapters may also be helpful to athletes competing in other sports or different situations. For example, you may be a swimmer who competes only in local galas, so the advice given to the travelling athlete may seem to be of no interest to you. However, if you go on a skiing holiday this advice, including guidance on exercising in the cold and at altitude, could well add to the enjoyment of your holiday – just have a look.

I hope you enjoy reading this book, that you find it informative and practical, and that you discover it is possible to 'Eat well, perform better'.

Jane Griffin
Accredited Sports Dietitian

CHAPTER 1

Nutrition

The body needs oxygen, water and nutrients to survive: without oxygen, death occurs within minutes; without water, death will take a few days; and without nutrients, death will occur after a few weeks. Until such time as nutrients are sold in discrete, neat packages and food and supermarkets become a thing of the past, it is necessary to know how to build up a diet from food in order to meet the body's requirements for each individual nutrient. People eat food but need nutrients.

Nutrients and Their Main Functions	
Nutrient	*Function*
Carbohydrate	Major source of energy or fuel for the body.
Fat	Major source of stored energy in the body.
Protein	Material for growth and repair of the body; component of enzymes, hormones and antibodies; source of energy for the body.
Vitamins	Used in regulation of chemical processes; not a source of energy, but involved in energy release from food.
Minerals	Help control the composition of body fluids; essential components of enzymes and proteins such as haemoglobin. Constituents of bones and teeth.

ENERGY

Introduction

It is commonly believed that energy is good and calories are bad or even fattening. This is a myth. In fact calories or more correctly kilocalories (kcal) are just a way of measuring energy. The metric equivalents are joules and kilojoules (multiplying kilocalories by 4.184, or 4.2 for convenience, converts them to kilojoules). Using kilojoules is more scientifically correct but kilocalories are more popular with the general public.

The human body is like a car and, as such, needs a source of fuel or energy in order to function properly. Individual energy requirements depend on a number of factors, based mainly on energy expenditure. There are four components of energy expenditure: basal metabolic rate (BMR); thermic effect of food (TEF); adaptive thermogenesis (AT); and physical activity.

Basal Metabolic Rate (BMR)
The basal metabolic rate is the amount of energy needed when the body is fasting and at

Converting Between Calories and Joules		
1kcal	=	4.18kJ
239kcal	=	1,000kJ (1MJ)
1,000kcal	=	4,180kJ (4.18MJ)

complete rest. It is the energy required by the body to maintain all bodily functions such as respiration, circulation, metabolism and so on. It is related to age (decreasing with age), sex (it is lower in women because of a higher proportion of body fat) and body weight (it is higher with a greater proportion of muscle mass). BMR can account for 60 to 75 per cent of total energy expenditure in sedentary individuals.

Thermic Effect of Food (TEF)
The thermic effect of food is the amount of energy needed for digestion, absorption, metabolism and storage of food. It accounts for about 10 per cent of the 24-hour energy expenditure. TEF is affected by the calorie content and composition of a meal.

Adaptive Thermogenesis (AT)
Sometimes called arousal, adaptive thermogenesis is the energy needed in times of environmental and physiological stress, such as changes in outside temperature. This is a very small component of total energy expenditure.

Physical Activity
Physical activity can be the most variable component of energy expenditure. A sedentary person may only expend 100kcal in activity during a day, whereas an elite athlete in hard training could expend 2,000kcal or more per day.

Energy Storage in the Body

There are three major energy stores in the body. The largest and most variable store is body fat (adipose tissue). Carbohydrate is stored in the liver and muscles as glycogen. Protein is stored primarily in muscle, but also in other tissues as well.

Calculating Basal Metabolic Rate (BMR)		
BMR (MJ/day)		
Age	*BMR (males)*	*BMR (females)*
10–17 years	0.074W + 2.754	0.056W + 2.898
18–29 years	0.063W + 2.896	0.062W + 2.036
30–59 years	0.048W + 3.653	0.034W + 3.538
60–74 years	0.0499W + 2.930	0.0386W + 2.875
75+ years	0.0350W + 3.434	0.041W + 2.610
BMR (kcal/day)		
Age	*BMR (males)*	*BMR (females)*
10–17 years	17.7W + 657	13.4W + 692
18–29 years	15.1W + 692	14.8W + 487
30–59 years	11.5W + 873	8.3W + 846
60–74 years	11.9W + 700	9.2W + 687
75+ years	8.4W + 821	9.8W + 624

W = body weight (kg)
Reference: Schofield W.N., Schofield C., James W.P.T. 'Basal metabolic rate – review and prediction' *Hum Nutr: Clin Nutr* (1985) 39 (suppl), pp 1–96.

Energy in Food

The energy to meet these requirements comes from the diet. Food is digested and absorbed, and then metabolized to release energy which the body can use. The same weight of different nutrients will provide different amounts of energy. Water, of course, has no calorific value.

- Protein: 4kcal per g (17kJ per g).
- Fat: 9kcal per g (37kJ per g).
- Carbohydrate: 4kcal per g (17kJ per g).
- Alcohol: 7kcal per g (29kJ per g).

Most foods are a mixture of these nutrients so that the total energy value of a food is the sum of the energy from each of the nutrients. However the proportions vary: foods may be mostly fat (for example butter, margarine and vegetable oils) or carbohydrate (for example sugar and glucose) or somewhere between. No food is predominantly protein. The more fat that is present in a food, the greater the total number of calories.

CARBOHYDRATES

The majority of carbohydrates in the diet come from plants, an exception being milk. Carbohydrates are the most important source of energy in the diet, being the primary energy source for exercising muscles, the brain and central nervous system. Indeed the brain needs 6g of glucose per hour or 144g of glucose per day, equivalent to approximately 600kcal per day, in order to function. Carbohydrates are classified according to their structure into 'simple' or 'complex' carbohydrates. Simple

---

Carbohydrate Facts

Simple Carbohydrates or Sugars

Name	Food Source	General Information
Glucose	Fruits, honey	Main source of energy in the body. Unique energy source for the brain.
Fructose	Fruits and fruit juices, honey	Directly absorbed and metabolized in the liver.
Galactose	Milk, yoghurt and milk products	Converted in the liver to glucose.
Sucrose	Table sugar	Important energy source, broken down in digestion to glucose and fructose. Used as a sweetener in a wide range of foods.
Lactose	Milk, milk products	Broken down in digestion to galactose and glucose.
Maltose	Beer, malted foods and some breakfast cereals	Broken down in digestion to glucose.

Complex Carbohydrates or Starches

Name	Food Source	General Information
Starch	Rice, bread, pasta, sweetcorn, pulses, potatoes and breakfast cereals	Broken down in digestion to maltose and then glucose.
Glycogen	Animal muscle and liver	Storage form of carbohydrate in muscle and liver. Stores are depleted by the time meat, fish or poultry are eaten.

Sources of Carbohydrate

Breakfast cereals

Bread

Crispbreads, waterbiscuits, oatcakes and rice cakes

Pasta

Rice

Noodles

Potatoes

Popcorn (sugared – buttered popcorn has a high fat content)

Pizza bases, preferably deep pan, though the topping can push up the fat content

Beans (baked, butter, red kidney etc.), peas, lentils, sweetcorn, pearl barley

Root vegetables – carrots, parsnips, swedes, beetroot

Fruit (all sorts) – fresh, dried, canned

Cereal bars, breakfast bars and squares (be careful: some have quite high fat contents)

Jam, marmalade, honey, fruit spreads

Savoury snacks

Biscuits

Cakes

Puddings

Yoghurt

Sweetened soft drinks

Fruit juice

Chocolate bars (be careful: many have high fat contents)

Sugar confectionery

Sugar

Sports drinks

Carbohydrate supplements (drinks, bars, gels, powders etc.)

---

carbohydrates or sugars are found in fruits, milk, vegetables, sugar cane and sugar beet and honey. Complex carbohydrates are the starches and fibrous materials found in bread, rice, cereals, pasta, potatoes and peas, beans and lentils (collectively called 'legumes' and when dried called 'pulses').

Although the general public is being encouraged to increase their carbohydrate consumption, many people do not see increasing the proportion of bread, rice, pasta and potatoes in the diet as a desirable dietary change. These foods are viewed, incorrectly, as high in calories and therefore unhelpful in weight control.

Dietary Fibre

Scientists are encouraging the term 'non-starch polysaccharides' to be used in place of 'dietary fibre' but like the use of calories rather than joules, the general public still prefers the term dietary fibre. Indeed, nutritional information on food packaging uses the term 'fibre'. Fibre occurs naturally in all plant foods (cereals, legumes, vegetables, fruits, nuts and seeds) as an integral structural component of the cell walls. It is made up of a varied group of compounds including cellulose, gums, hemicellulose, lignin and pectin. Officially dietary fibre is not classed as a nutrient as its beneficial effects actually come about because it is *not* digested and absorbed in the gut.

Fibre is classified as 'soluble' and 'insoluble', with different beneficial properties for each type of fibre. Soluble fibre is found in oats, legumes, leafy vegetables and certain fruits such as apples. It is believed to help in reducing blood cholesterol levels and also to help in slowing down the absorption of glucose in the blood in some types of diabetes. Insoluble fibre is found in cereals and cereal products. It has a role to play in maintaining a healthy gut, primarily by helping to prevent constipation and the resulting bowel disorders. High fibre foods are also by their nature filling foods but without providing excessive calories. For those who need to lose or maintain a low weight for competition, use of these bulky foods can be particularly useful in helping to limit food intake while keeping hunger at bay. However for those with high carbohydrate requirements, including a large proportion of fibre-rich carbohydrate foods can make the diet very bulky and filling. This can have the effect of limiting overall food intake with the result that daily energy and nutrient requirements, including carbohydrate requirements, are not met.

Glycaemic Index

There is still a widespread belief that simple carbohydrates or sugars are digested and absorbed more rapidly than the complex or starchy types. This has led to many people making inappropriate food choices, particularly for pre-event meals and snacks (*see* Chapter 4). The glycaemic index (GI) factor is a ranking of foods from 0 to 100 based on the rate at which a food raises the blood glucose level. Foods with a low GI factor cause a slow rise in blood glucose level, whereas foods with a high GI factor cause a rapid rise. Looking at the GI factor of commonly consumed foods, it becomes apparent that sugars are not necessarily absorbed more rapidly than starches. A word of caution here, as the figures relate to the food when eaten alone. The GI factor can change when other foods are consumed at the same time. For instance, the consumption of fat slows the rate of gastric emptying and consequently alters the GI effect.

The Starch Versus Sugar Debate

The energy contribution from sugars and starches is much the same and digestion ultimately reduces both primarily to glucose. So is there a place for both in the diet, or is sugar still the enemy?

'Starchy foods are good sources of various nutrients.'
It is true that potatoes contain vitamin C and bread contains B vitamins, calcium and iron. However, sugar is pure carbohydrate and is therefore a useful energy source. Sugar is also an ingredient in many foods that not only provide nutrients but also add variety to the diet.

'Starchy foods provide bulk without excessive calories.'
This is true if the natural fibre content is retained. In some situations, adding bulk to the diet will be an advantage but this is not always the case.

'Starchy foods are a good source of fibre.'
This is true; however the fibre may have been removed in processing.

'Starchy foods do not encourage tooth decay.'
The only fact that nobody seems to dispute is that a high sugar diet can increase the risk of tooth decay. Foods containing starch, particularly those with a high GI factor, may be easily broken down by bacteria in the mouth to produce acid, which also increases the risk of tooth decay. The impact of these carbohydrates on tooth decay depends on a number of factors including the type of food, the frequency of eating, general oral hygiene and use of fluoride.

'Sugar causes illnesses such as diabetes, cancer and heart disease.'
Sugar does not cause diabetes. Diabetes occurs when the body is not producing

How Different Foods Affect Blood Sugar Levels

Type of food	Low GI	Moderate GI	High GI
Drinks	Sugar free drinks	Sports drinks; Fanta™, cola	Lucozade™; glucose drinks
Cereals	All Bran™; muesli; porridge; Special K™; Sultana Bran; Fruit & Fibre type; oat and wheat flakes	Shreddies™; Sustain; grapenuts; Cheerios; Branbuds	Cornflakes; Cocopops; Rice Krispies; Weetabix; puffed rice; puffed wheat; Shredded Wheat
Bread, biscuits and cake	Heavy grain bread such as granary/ multi-grain; pitta bread; chapatis; fruit loaf; sponge cake*; banana cake*	Fibre-enriched white; bread; Ryvita™; oatmeal biscuits; shortbread*; muesli bars*; flapjacks*; croissants*; muffins; digestive biscuits	Brown bread; wholemeal bread; white bread; french sticks; bagels; crumpets; morning coffee biscuits; water biscuits; puffed crispbreads; rice cakes
Potatoes, rice and pasta	Yams; sweet potatoes; basmati rice; noodles; pasta (most types)	New potatoes; boiled potatoes; macaroni	Instant potato; mashed potato; jacket potatoes; chips*; instant rice; brown/white rice
Fruit and vegetables	Apples; dried apricots; banana; cherries; cantaloupe melon; grapefruit; grapes; kiwi; mango; orange; peach (canned and fresh); pear; plum; fruit cocktail; apple, orange, grapefruit or pineapple juice (small glass); carrots, peas, sweetcorn	Apricots (canned); pineapple; papaya; squash; sultanas; raisins; pineapple	Parsnips; pumpkins; swede; broad beans; watermelon
Legumes and grains	Baked beans; butter beans; black eyed beans; chick peas; haricot beans; kidney beans; lentils; soya beans; pearl barley; buckwheat; bulgar wheat	Couscous; cornmeal; millet	Tapioca
Snacks	Most chocolate*; popcorn; crisps*; peanuts*	Some chocolate bars such as Mars bars™; taco shells	Jelly babies/beans; corn chips
Sugars	Fructose; lactose	Honey; sucrose	Glucose
Dairy products	Low fat ice-cream; milk; yoghurt	Full fat ice cream*	

* Foods containing relatively high amounts of fat.

Table reproduced by kind permission of Beta Cell Dietitians, Chelsea and Westminster Healthcare NHS Trust.

enough insulin. Sugar does not cause cancer or heart disease.

'Sugar causes obesity.'

Sugar does not cause obesity. Sugars and starches stimulate a feedback mechanism in the body that helps to control appetite and so reduces the risk of overeating. (The same cannot be said of fat.)

FAT

Dietary fat is a vital nutrient and should be included in the diet. Although a large percentage of the population consumes too much fat, it is both unnecessary and unhealthy to try to exclude fat totally from the diet. Fat is an important source of energy and the fat in adipose tissue not only acts as an energy store but also provides insulation for the body and support and cushioning for the vital organs such as the liver and kidneys. Fat is needed as the carrier for the fat-soluble vitamins A, D, E and K and to help in their absorption. The body also has a requirement for essential fatty acids. These are needed for good health yet the body cannot make them and must rely on the diet to provide them. Fats in the diet are responsible for much of the flavour, smell and texture of foods and therefore have a key role in maintaining the palatability of the diet.

However, since fat is a concentrated source of energy, a high intake can lead to obesity and its associated health risks, including heart disease.

The Different Types of Fats in the Diet

Dietary fats are made up of triglycerides which all have the same structure: a backbone of glycerol with three fatty acids attached in an 'E' shape. The fatty acids may be saturated, monounsaturated or polyunsaturated. Dietary

---

> **Sources of Fat**
>
> **Visible fats:** butter, margarine, ghee, oils, lard, suet, dripping, cream; fat on meat, poultry skin.
> **Invisible fats:** fat is present in all but the very lean cuts of meat; cheese (especially full fat); whole milk (silver or gold top); eggs; meat products (such as pies, pasties, sausages, burgers, pâté and salami, tinned meats); chips, crisps and roast potatoes; fried food and pastry; nuts, olives, avocado pears; some types of cakes and biscuits; creamy puddings and cheesecakes; mayonnaise, salad cream and creamy sauces; peanut butter; chocolate, toffee, fudge.

---

fats are made up of different mixtures of these types of fatty acids.

Fats containing a high proportion of saturated fatty acids tend to be solid at room temperature while those that contain high proportions of unsaturated fatty acids are usually liquid at room temperature.

Essential Fatty Acids

There are two families of essential fatty acids which the diet must supply, the omega-6

> **Fat Facts**
>
> | Type of fat | Source |
> | --- | --- |
> | Saturated | Mainly animal origin: dairy products, meat and poultry; also coconut oil, palm oil. |
> | Monounsaturated | Olive oil; peanuts; almonds; avocado pears; rapeseed oil. |
> | Polyunsaturated | Sunflower, corn, soybean, cottonseed and safflower oils; oily fish and lean meat. |

Sources of Essential Fatty Acids

Omega-6 family: lean meat; sunflower, corn and soya oil; margarines made from sunflower, corn or soya oil; rapeseed oil.
Omega-3 family: oily fish; soya bean and rapeseed oil; green vegetables.

---

family (linolenic acid) and omega-3 family (alpha linolenic acid). They are vital for the development of cell membranes and are also involved in the regulation of immune responses and blood clotting. Research suggests that they may help in the prevention of heart disease and strokes.

Cholesterol

Cholesterol is an essential part of cell membranes. It is involved in protecting nerve fibres and it plays a role in the production of vitamin D and certain hormones, including the sex hormones.

Dietary sources of cholesterol are of animal origin only, namely egg yolks, liver and kidney, fish roes and shellfish. However the main source of cholesterol in the blood is not directly from dietary cholesterol. Cholesterol is made in the liver and high intakes of saturated fats are associated with increased levels of blood cholesterol. A raised level of blood cholesterol is a risk indicator for heart disease.

Hydrogenated Fats and Trans Fatty Acids

Fats with a high proportion of polyunsaturated fatty acids tend to be liquid at room temperature and are also unstable and likely to turn rancid or go off. When these oils are used to make margarines and cooking fats, they have to be hardened or hydrogenated. This process not only converts some of the unsaturated fat into saturated fat but also changes the actual structure of the fatty acids to form trans fatty acids.

It is thought that trans fatty acids, like saturated fatty acids, may be a risk factor in heart disease. Although a Department of Health report on diet and prevention of heart disease recommended that intake should be limited to no more than the present intake of about 2 per cent of total energy or 5g per day, food labelling does not require the trans fatty acid content to be declared. Trans fatty acids occur naturally in the fat and milk of multi-stomached animals that chew the cud, such as cattle and sheep. However some research has suggested that these naturally occurring trans fatty acids do not present any problems.

The main sources of hydrogenated fat and therefore trans fatty acids in the diet are margarines, shortenings and products such as biscuits and pastries made using these ingredients.

PROTEIN

Protein is needed to build and maintain all the cells in the body, a unique function that no other nutrient can fulfil. Cells are constantly being replaced and an intake of protein is therefore needed on a daily basis. During periods of growth and development there is an additional need for protein. Children and adolescents will, therefore, have a proportionally greater requirement than adults.

Protein is essential in the actual structures of the body for the formation of muscle, bones, skin and hair. Functionally, it is involved in hormone and enzyme production. Antibodies, which fight off infections and diseases, are proteins. Haemoglobin, which is used to transport oxygen in the blood, is also protein in nature.

If carbohydrates and fats are not eaten in sufficient amounts, protein can be used to

Sources of Protein	
Animal sources	*Vegetable sources*
Meat	Beans, peas and lentils
Offal	Nuts and seeds
Poultry	Quorn, tofu
Fish, shellfish	Soya and soya milk
Eggs	Textured vegetable protein
Milk, cheese, yoghurt	Bread, potatoes, rice, pasta, cereals

Classification of Amino Acids	
Essential amino acids	*Non-essential amino acids*
Isoleucine	Alanine
Leucine	Arginine
Lysine	Asparagine
Methionine	Aspartic acid
Phenylalanine	Cysteine/cystine
Threonine	Glutamic acid
Tryptophan	Glutamine
Valine	Glycine
Histidine (in infants)	Proline
	Serine
	Tyrosine

meet energy demands. Protein cannot be stored for later use like carbohydrate and fat, so if more protein is consumed than the body needs for growth, maintenance and repair the excess protein is either broken down and used for energy or converted into fat and stored.

Amino Acids

Proteins are made up of amino acids linked together in long chains. The body needs twenty different amino acids for its structure and function. Eight of these amino acids are essential. They cannot be made by the body and must therefore be provided by the diet. The remaining amino acids are non-essential and can be made from other amino acids. In the case of cysteine and tyrosine these amino acids can only be made from the essential amino acids methionine and phenylalanine.

The nutritional value of a protein depends on its ability to provide the quality and quantity of the essential amino acids that the body needs. Generally proteins from animal sources, such as meat, fish, eggs, milk and cheese are good sources of essential amino acids. Vegetable sources of protein tend to be low in one or more of these essential amino acids. Wheat is low in lysine while beans are low in methionine, but a meal of baked beans on toast would provide all the essential amino acids. It is therefore particularly important that vegetarians eat a wide range of vegetable sources of protein to ensure an adequate intake of all the essential amino acids.

Too Much Protein in the Diet

High-protein diets increase the workload of the kidneys because of the extra nitrogen that must be excreted (*see* Chapter 2). This does not seem to be a problem in otherwise healthy people except possibly for physically active individuals who already have increased fluid losses through sweating.

In the past, high-protein diets have been linked with an increased loss of calcium in the urine. This could be a potential problem, particularly for women because of the potential to speed up the development of osteoporosis or brittle bone disease. However the link is with purified protein supplements rather than with food. Protein-rich foods that are good sources of calcium are also good sources of phosphorus, and the presence of phosphorus or phosphate appears to inhibit the calcium loss.

VITAMINS AND MINERALS

Vitamins and minerals are found naturally in food and are vital in the maintenance of all body functions. They help to maintain health and prevent disease. Different foods supply different vitamins and minerals in varying amounts and therefore a wide range of foods must be included in a diet if requirements for these essential nutrients are to be met. In 1991, the United Kingdom Department of Health published guidelines for the intake of nutrients using a new term, the Reference Nutrient Intake (RNI). (Department of Health Report on Health and Social Subjects No. 41 *Dietary Reference Values for Food Energy and Nutrients for the United Kingdom* (HMSO, 1991).) The RNI was defined as the amount of a nutrient that is sufficient for almost every individual, even a person who has high needs for the nutrient. This level of intake is, therefore, considerably higher than most people need. If an individual consumes the RNI of a nutrient, that person is most unlikely to be deficient in that nutrient.

Vitamins

Vitamins do not provide energy, although some are involved in the release of energy from food. They are required by the body in very small amounts compared to the requirements for carbohydrate and protein. Vitamins, with the exception of vitamin D, cannot be made in the body and must be provided by the diet. They are classified as fat-soluble (vitamins A, D, E and K) or water-soluble (vitamin C and the B-complex vitamins). Fat-soluble vitamins are stored in the body until required. Water-soluble vitamins are not stored in the body and must be provided by the diet on a regular basis. An intake of water-soluble vitamins in excess of requirements is usually excreted in the urine.

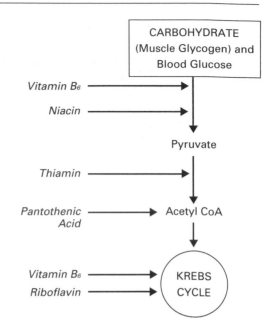

Use of B Vitamins in Energy Release from Carbohydrate.

Vitamin A

Major food sources   Vitamin A is found in animal foods as retinol. Plant foods contain beta-carotene, the precursor of vitamin A. Richest sources of vitamin A are fish liver oils (cod liver oil) and animal liver (lamb, calf and pig). Good sources of vitamin A include oily fish (mackerel, herring, tuna, sardines and salmon), egg yolk, full fat milk, butter, cheese and fortified margarine. Good sources of beta-carotene are fruit and vegetables, especially yellow (carrots, apricots), dark green (spinach, watercress and broccoli) and red (tomatoes and red peppers) fruit and vegetables.

Main functions   Essential for healthy skin. Maintains healthy mucous membranes in the throat and nose. Protects against poor vision in dim light. Antioxidant properties.

Deficiency   Very rare in the UK. In third world countries deficiency is a major cause of blindness.

Requirement RNI 700µg per day for adult men; 600µg per day for adult women.

Excessive intakes Regular intakes of retinol should not exceed 9,000µg for adult men, 7,500µg for adult women or 3,300µg for pregnant women. Women who are or might become pregnant are advised by the Department of Health not to take vitamin A supplements or eat liver because of an increased risk of birth defects.

Vitamin B₁ (Thiamin)

Major food sources Cereal products such as breakfast cereals, bread, pasta and rice, lean pork and peas, beans and lentils.

Main functions Release of energy from carbohydrate. Required for normal functioning of nerves, brain and muscles.

Deficiency Very rare in the UK. Causes beri-beri which affects the heart and nervous system.

Requirement RNI 1.0mg per day for adult men; 0.8mg per day for adult women. (This is dependent on the energy content of the diet: the RNI is set at 0.4mg per 1,000kcal for most groups of people.)

Excessive intakes Chronic intakes in excess of 3g per day are toxic in adults.

Vitamin B₂ (Riboflavin)

Major food sources Milk, egg yolks, liver, kidneys, cheese, wholemeal bread and cereals and green vegetables. Sensitive to light.

Main functions Release of energy from carbohydrate, fat and protein.

Deficiency Sores in the corners of the mouth. Severe deficiency is unlikely in the UK.

Requirement RNI 1.3mg per day for adult men; 1.1mg per day for adult women.

Excessive intakes Absorption of riboflavin in the intestine is limited so toxic effects are unlikely.

Niacin (Nicotinic Acid, Nicotinamide, Vitamin B₃)

Major food sources Meat, poultry, fortified breakfast cereals, white flour and bread, yeast extracts.

Main functions Release of energy from protein, fat and carbohydrate.

Deficiency Rare.

Requirement RNI 17mg per day for adult men; 13mg per day for adult women.

Excessive intakes Very high intakes in the region of 3 to 6g per day may cause liver damage.

Vitamin B₆ (Pyridoxine)

Major food sources Meat, particularly beef and poultry, fish, wholemeal bread and fortified breakfast cereals.

Main functions Needed for protein metabolism, central nervous system functioning, haemoglobin production and antibody formation.

Deficiency Deficiency signs are rare.

Requirement RNI 1.4mg per day for adult men; 1.2 mg per day for adult women.

Excessive intakes High intakes have been associated with impaired function of sensory nerves. Amounts involved have varied from 50mg per day to 2 to 7g per day.

Vitamin B₁₂ (Cyanocobalamin)

Major food sources Found only in food of animal origin (liver, kidney, meat, oily fish, milk, cheese and eggs). Some breakfast cereals are fortified with vitamin B₁₂. Some vegetarian foods are also fortified, for example soya protein, soya milks and yeast extract.

Main functions Red blood cell formation, maintenance of nervous system and protein metabolism.

Deficiency Pernicious anaemia (blood disorder).

Requirement RNI 1.5µg per day for adult men and women.

Excessive intakes   Excreted in the urine and therefore not dangerous.

Folic Acid (Folates)
Major food sources   Liver, kidney, green leafy vegetables, wholegrain cereals, fortified breakfast cereals and breads, eggs, pulses, bananas and orange juice.
Main functions   Red and white blood cell formation in bone marrow. Essential for growth. Protects against neural tube defects (spina bifida) pre-conceptually and in early pregnancy.
Deficiency   Megaloblastic anaemia (blood disorder).
Requirement   RNI 200µg per day for adults. Women who might become pregnant and pregnant women during the first twelve weeks of pregnancy are recommended to take an extra 400µg per day.
Excessive intakes   Dangers of toxicity are very low.

Biotin and Pantothenic Acid
Major food sources   Widespread in food.
Main functions   Release of energy from fat, carbohydrate and protein.
Deficiency   Unlikely.
Requirement   None set.
Excessive intakes   No danger.

Vitamin C
Major food sources   Fruit and vegetables especially blackcurrants, strawberries and citrus fruit, raw peppers, tomatoes and green leafy vegetables. Potatoes also provide vitamin C and this contribution may be significant because of the quantity eaten in the average UK diet.
Main functions   Required for healthy skin, blood vessels, gums and teeth, wound healing, iron absorption and formation of antibodies. Important antioxidant.
Deficiency   Scurvy. Mild deficiency leads to tiredness, bleeding gums, delayed wound healing and lowered resistance to infection.
Requirement   RNI 40mg per day for adults.
Excessive intakes   Intakes at levels of twenty times the RNI or more have been associated with diarrhoea and increased risk of oxalate stones in the kidney.

Vitamin D (Cholecalciferol)
Major food sources   Fortified margarines and spreads, fortified breakfast cereals, oily fish, egg yolks, full fat milk and dairy products. The main source of vitamin D is the action of UV light on the skin.
Main function   Absorption of calcium and its utilisation in the body particularly the mineralization of bones and teeth.
Deficiency   Loss of calcium from the bones, causing rickets in young children and osteo-malacia particularly in women of child-bearing age.
Requirement   No dietary source needed for adults provided that skin is exposed to sunlight (RNI for adults aged 65 and over is 10µg per day.)
Excessive intakes   Toxicity is rare in adults.

Vitamin E
Major food sources   Vegetable oils, seeds, nuts (especially peanuts), wheat germ, whole-meal bread and cereals, green plants, milk and milk products and egg yolks.
Main functions   Powerful antioxidant, pro-tecting body tissues against free radical damage.
Deficiency   None except in very exceptional circumstances.
Requirement   No RNI set: 4mg per day for adult men and 3mg per day for adult women is considered adequate.
Excessive intakes   Toxicity extremely rare.

Vitamin K
Major food sources   Dark green leafy vegetables, margarines and vegetable oils, milk

and liver. Also synthesized by bacteria in the gut.

Main functions   Blood clotting.

Deficiency   Rare in adults.

Requirement   No RNI set but 1µg per kg per day is considered both safe and adequate.

Excessive intakes   Natural K vitamins seem free from toxic side effects, even up to one hundred times the safe intake. Synthetic forms may not have such a margin of safety.

Minerals

Some minerals are required in relatively large amounts. These include calcium (which makes up 2 per cent of the total body weight of an adult), chloride, magnesium, phosphorus, potassium and sodium. Other minerals are also required but in such small amounts that they are known as 'trace elements'. These include iodine, which accounts for just 0.00004 per cent of the total body weight of an adult, chromium, copper, fluoride, iron, manganese, molybdenum, selenium and zinc.

Calcium

Major food sources   Milk, cheese and yoghurt (low fat and full fat), tinned sardines and pilchards (from the edible bones), dark green leafy vegetables, pulses (including baked beans), white flour and white bread (fortified) and hard water.

Main functions   Essential for strong and healthy bones and teeth. Important in blood clotting. Essential for nerve and muscle function.

Deficiency   Causes problems with bones, which may become brittle and break easily (osteoporosis or brittle bone disease). Good calcium intakes in childhood and adolescence are vital to help build up calcium in the bones and to protect against osteoporosis in later life.

Requirement   RNI 700mg per day for adult men and women. Vitamin D is essential for the absorption of calcium.

Excessive intakes   Calcium toxicity is virtually unknown. The body adapts to high intakes by reducing the amount that is absorbed.

Phosphorus

Major food sources   Present in all plant and animal foods except fats and sugars.

Main functions   Essential for the formation of bones and teeth. Involved in many metabolic reactions.

Deficiency   Unknown.

Requirement   RNI 550mg per day for adult men and women.

Excessive intakes   Not known in adults.

Magnesium

Major food sources   Present in most foods, particularly cereals, vegetables (especially dark green leafy vegetables) and fruit.

Main functions   Energy production, nerve and muscle function and bone structure.

Deficiency   Body is very efficient at regulating magnesium content so deficiencies are rare. Deficiencies are usually caused by severe diarrhoea or excessive losses in urine resulting from the use of diuretics.

Requirements   RNI 300mg per day for adult men; 270mg per day for adult women.

Excessive intakes   No evidence that high intakes are harmful if kidney function is normal.

Sodium and Chloride

Major food sources   As sodium chloride (salt). About 15 to 20 per cent of sodium chloride in the diet is naturally present in food, 15 to 29 per cent is added in cooking or to the food once served and 60 to 79 per cent is added during food processing or manufacture. Foods high in sodium chloride include ham, bacon, smoked fish, foods canned in brine, cheese, butter, salted nuts and biscuits and yeast extract. Significant contributions are also made by bread, breakfast cereal, ready meats, canned meats, savoury snacks, soups and sauces consumed on a regular basis.

Main functions Regulation of body water content, maintenance of acid-base balance, blood volume and blood pressure and nerve and muscle function.

Deficiency Unlikely in normal circumstances.

Requirement RNI 1,600mg per day for sodium and 2,500mg per day for chloride for adult men and women.

Excessive intakes Habitually high intakes of salt may be linked with the development of high blood pressure or hypertension.

Potassium

Major food sources Present in all foods except fats, oils and sugar. Particularly good sources are fruits (bananas and oranges), vegetables, potatoes, coffee, tea and cocoa.

Main functions Regulation of fluid balance in conjunction with sodium. Potassium maintains water inside the cells (intracellular fluid) and sodium maintains water outside the cells (extracellular fluid). Also nerve and muscle function.

Deficiency Unlikely. Can result from severe diarrhoea and vomiting.

Requirements RNI 3,500mg per day for adult men and women.

Excessive intakes Toxicity only likely to occur by supplementation.

Iron

Major food sources Liver, lean meat (especially red meat), kidney, heart, shellfish and egg yolks. Wholegrain cereals, dried pulses and dried fruit contain iron but it is less well absorbed than iron from animal foods. Some breakfast cereals are fortified with iron. Vitamin C helps the absorption of iron from plant foods.

Main function Part of haemoglobin in red blood cells which carries oxygen to all parts of the body.

Deficiency Low haemoglobin levels cause tiredness and fatigue and ultimately iron deficiency anaemia. Iron deficiency is one of the commonest nutritional deficiencies in developed and developing countries. As many as one in three women of child-bearing age in the UK is iron deficient.

Requirement RNI 8.7mg per day for adult men; 14.8mg for women (11 to 50 plus years) per day. RNI for women is higher to make up for iron losses due to monthly periods.

Excessive intakes No risk from normal foods other than in people with rare metabolic disorders.

Zinc

Major food sources Red meat, liver, shellfish (especially oysters), dairy products and eggs. Whole grain cereals, bread and pulses contain zinc but it is less well absorbed from these sources.

Main functions Part of many enzymes needed for a variety of body functions, involved in energy production, aiding wound healing, in development of the body's immune system (antioxidant function) and in insulin production.

Deficiency Insufficient zinc can slow down growth and development. It also delays wound healing and may impair immune function.

Requirement RNI 9.5mg per day for adult men; 9.5mg per day for adult women.

Excessive intakes Acute ingestion of 2g of zinc produces nausea and vomiting. Long term intakes of 50mg per day interfere with copper metabolism.

Copper

Major food sources Present in trace quantities in many foods.

Main functions Part of many enzyme systems, particularly those involved in metabolism and antioxidant function.
Deficiency Copper deficiency may have a role in the development of heart disease but more research is needed.
Requirement RNI 1.2mg per day for adult men and women.
Excessive intakes High intakes are toxic but these occur only in abnormal circumstances such as contamination of water.

Selenium
Major food sources Whole grain cereals, meat, fish and shellfish, milk and egg yolks and Brazil nuts. The selenium content of food is dependent on the amount of selenium present in the soil where it is grown.
Main function Powerful antioxidant (protects cell membranes).
Deficiency No clinical condition is associated with a dietary deficiency but there is a possible link with the development of heart disease.
Requirement RNI 75µg per day for adult men; 60µg per day for adult women.
Excessive intakes High levels (in excess of 1mg) are known to be toxic and an upper limit of 6µg per kg per day for adults has been set.

Fluoride
Major food sources Drinking water with a high natural or added fluoride level, fluoride toothpaste, fish and tea.
Main function Bone and tooth mineralization and helping in the prevention of tooth decay.
Deficiency Increased susceptibility to tooth decay and lack of bone strength.
Requirement No RNI set.
Excessive intakes Causes mottling of teeth.

Iodine
Major food sources The only naturally rich source is seafood. Other sources are milk and milk products and iodised salt.
Main function Functioning of the thyroid and formation of thyroid hormones.
Deficiency Resulting deficiency of thyroid hormone leads to a low metabolic rate and lethargy.
Requirement RNI 140µg per day for adult men and women.
Excessive intakes Not usually a problem.

Manganese
Major food sources Tea.
Main function Component of many enzymes.
Deficiency Unobserved except in experimental studies.
Requirement No RNI set but safe intakes are believed to lie above 1.4mg per day for adults.
Excessive intakes One of the least toxic elements. Excess intakes are quickly excreted.

Chromium
Major food sources Meat, whole grain cereals, legumes, nuts and brewer's yeast.
Main function Formation of insulin and lipoprotein metabolism.
Deficiency Unlikely on a normal mixed diet.
Requirements No RNI set but safe intakes are believed to lie above 25µg per day for adults.

Molybdenum
Major food sources Trace amounts found in many foods.
Main function Enzyme function.
Deficiency Reported on very low intakes (25µg per day) where the typical UK diet provides a mean of 128µg per day
Requirements No RNI set but safe intakes are believed to lie between 50 and 400µg per day.

Vitamin and Mineral Supplements

A balanced diet should provide all the vitamins and minerals required but in some situations this is not possible and a supplement is needed. Natural and synthetic vitamin supplements do the same job, but natural ones tend to be more expensive. In most cases a supplement that provides no more than the RNI in one day's dosage is all that is needed. A supplement *adds* to what the diet is already providing and so large doses are not likely to be necessary. If supplements are used they should be taken regularly and only in the recommended daily dosage.

ANTIOXIDANT NUTRIENTS

Antioxidants are a group of vitamins, minerals and plant substances (variously called phytochemicals, bioactive compounds or phytoprotectants) which have an important role in protecting the body against the effects of highly active substances in the body called free radicals. Free radicals are produced as a by-product of reactions in the body, a perfectly normal process. However production is increased by exposure to various environmental pollutants such as cigarette smoke, car fumes and excessive exposure to sunlight.

Free radicals have the potential to damage cells in the body and the genetic material contained in cells unless they are mopped up by antioxidants and neutralized. Damage to cells by free radicals is thought to be partly to blame for chronic diseases such as cancer and heart disease.

The antioxidant vitamins are vitamin A and its precursor betacarotene (and probably other carotenoids), vitamin C and vitamin E (often referred to as the 'ACE vitamins'). Minerals with antioxidant properties include zinc, copper and selenium. Phytochemicals found particularly in fruit and vegetables and believed to have antioxidant properties include lycopene (tomatoes), saponins (onions), allicin (garlic) and indoles (broccoli, cabbage and Brussels sprouts).

WATER

Up to 55 to 65 per cent of the adult body is made up of water, equivalent in volume to ten gallons or forty litres. As so much of the body is water, it is not surprising that it plays a key role in sustaining life. Water is an integral part of all body cells and a constituent of all bodily fluids. It is therefore vital in transporting nutrients and oxygen around the body and getting rid of waste matter via the kidneys in urine. The sweat mechanism enables the maintenance of body temperature. Water is needed for many of the chemical reactions that take place during digestion, to keep joints and the eyes well lubricated, to facilitate swallowing and to help in the transport of sound through the inner ear. Water is needed to maintain blood volume and pressure and it also aids respiration.

How Much Water is Needed?

It is generally agreed that healthy adults need between two and three litres of fluid each day (more when exercising or during hot weather). This is approximately equivalent to the amount that is lost each day. With so many important functions dependent on water, it is vital that a constant level of hydration is maintained. The body does not store water in the way that fat and carbohydrate can be stored so a regular intake is important. As a very general rule of thumb, urination every two to four hours is probably a sign that sufficient fluids are being consumed.

The body loses water through sweating, during respiration when water vapour is lost

Patrick Rafter takes a drink between games at the 1997 US Open.

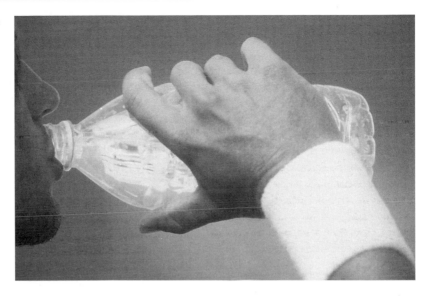

on expiration and in the elimination of urine and faeces. Water loss can increase considerably in extreme situations such as vomiting, diarrhoea, fever and intensive exercise. Water gains come from what is eaten and drunk and from the metabolism of nutrients. Metabolism of a 3,000kcal mixed diet will yield approximately 400ml of water a day. Water in food provides about 500ml to 800ml per day.

Recommended Daily Intake of Water	
Age	*Amount ml/kg body weight*
1 day	60
2 days	90
3 days	120
9 months	135
12 months	92
2 years	83
4 years	66
8 years	62
12 years	58
20 years	35
50 years	35
65 years	30

Water Content of Selected Foods	
Type of food	*Water content g per 100g edible portion)*
Bananas	75
Butter, margarine	16
Cheese	36
Chestnuts	52
Chicken	75
Chips	57
Crisps	2
Dried dates	12
Eggs	75
Lettuce	95
Low fat spread	50
Melon	92
Milk	88
Oranges	86
Peanuts	6
Peas	75
Potatoes	79
Soft drinks	90
Tomatoes	93
Vegetable oil	0
White fish	82
Yoghurt	77

Too Little Water

The body cannot survive many days without water. If water losses are not replaced through food and fluids, the body tries to conserve water through a variety of mechanisms. Progression of dehydration becomes apparent through the following sequence:

(1) intense thirst, generalized discomfort, loss of appetite;
(2) fatigue, nausea, emotional behaviour;
(3) headaches and tingling in the hands, arms and legs;
(4) increase in body temperature, pulse and rate of breathing;
(5) weakness, mental confusion, muscle spasms;
(6) decreased blood volume and blood circulation;
(7) cracked skin and halt to urine production;
(8) death.

Unfortunately the thirst mechanism is not a good indicator of dehydration. The sensation of thirst is felt sometime after the body has started to become dehydrated. Advice is therefore to top-up fluid levels constantly throughout the day in order to remain well hydrated (*see* Chapter 4).

Too Much Water

Oedema is caused by the accumulation of excessive water in the tissues of the body. This is not due to excessive intakes of fluid but to medical conditions such as heart failure, kidney disease, severe burns or an inability to regulate sodium.

Water intoxication results when water intake occurs faster than the body can form urine. This can happen in the clinical situation when, for example, a patient is given excessive amounts of intravenous fluid. It does not normally occur in non-clinical situations.

ALCOHOL

Alcohol is made by the fermentation of yeast, water and carbohydrates. For example, sugar in grapes ferments to make wine, and beer is produced by the fermentation of malted barley and hops.

The Effect of Alcohol Consumption

About 20 per cent of the alcohol contained in a drink is absorbed rapidly through the stomach, and the remainder is absorbed through the small intestine. Once absorbed into the blood, it circulates to all parts of the body where it acts both as a stimulant and a depressant. It stimulates the heart to beat faster and the blood vessels to widen, causing flushing and a pleasant feeling of warmth. However, this feeling of warmth is superficial as blood is diverted to the skin so that the body actually loses heat. This is why alcohol should never be given to someone who is suffering from exposure to the cold.

Alcohol also stimulates the gastric juices, so acting as an appetizer. It has a depressant effect on the brain and central nervous system, causing problems with co-ordination and balance. The staggering, clumsy drunk at a party is an all too familiar sight. Reaction times are slower and there is a loss of ability to judge distances. Apart from affecting intellectual and sexual performance, regular drinking in anything more than moderation can seriously damage the liver and heart.

The Fate of Alcohol

About 10 per cent of alcohol drunk is eliminated from the body through sweating, breathing and excretion via the kidneys in urine. The remaining 90 per cent is broken down at a fixed rate by the liver. Excessive intakes will therefore be stockpiled resulting in high levels of alcohol in the blood until the liver can metabolize it. The liver metabolizes alcohol at a set rate of about 1 unit (10ml alcohol) an hour.

Regular drinkers tolerate alcohol better than the occasional drinker does. This is because when alcohol reaches the liver it stimulates the production of the enzyme needed to break it down. The more that is drunk, the more the liver is stimulated to produce the enzyme. With time and regular drinking, a greater amount of alcohol will be required to reach the same state of intoxication. The liver has learnt to cope with the alcohol level and has built up tolerance, but this is also the time when liver damage can begin.

Energy is released with the breakdown of alcohol and this can be used immediately or stored as fat for use at a later date. However its use as a source of energy in exercise is limited.

Problems Linked with Alcohol Intake

Aside from the serious long-term problems of regular, addictive heavy intakes of alcohol, such as liver and heart disease and some forms of cancer, there are more common problems.

Weight Gain
An alcoholic drink is a concentrated source of calories. Anyone trying to lose weight would do well to steer away from alcoholic drinks of all kinds or at least restrict consumption.

- Half a pint of bitter contains 90kcal.
- An average glass of wine contains 75kcal.
- Half a pint of low alcohol lager contains 60kcal.
- A measure of spirits contains 50kcal.

Vitamins and Minerals
Alcoholic drinks contain negligible amounts of essential nutrients such as vitamins and minerals.

Ten large cans of beer are needed to reach the recommended daily intake of vitamin B_2 and significantly larger amounts are needed to reach an adequate intake of other vitamins. Excessive intake actually impairs the absorption of vitamin B_1, folic acid, vitamin B_{12} and vitamin C.

Hangovers
Hangovers are actually caused by the dehydrating effect of alcohol which acts as a diuretic, taking fluid from the body and increasing urine output. The non-alcoholic congeners that give flavour, smell and colour (where appropriate) to a drink also contribute to the symptoms of a hangover.

There are some simple steps that can be taken to prevent a hangover, apart from the obvious step of not drinking. Drink up to one litre of water either with the alcoholic drinks or before going to sleep. Keep water by the bedside in case of waking thirsty in the night. Failing this, drink water or fruit juice immediately on waking. Avoid alcoholic drinks with high congener levels such as port, brandy, whisky/whiskey, liqueurs, dark rum, dark beer and home-made wines.

Black coffee is not a wise 'morning after the night before' drink. Caffeine in coffee has a diuretic effect and will compound the dehydrating effect of alcohol. Decaffeinated coffee is fine. Aspirin is of little use as the headache is caused by dehydration not tension. It may also irritate an already sensitive stomach lining, which will not help the waves of nausea.

Women and Alcohol

Women break down alcohol at a slower rate than men do because, in general, they have smaller bodies with more fat and less fluid. The intoxicating effects for the same amount of alcohol are therefore apparent for longer. Women are more sensitive to alcohol at certain times in the menstrual cycle when hormone levels change.

High consumption of alcohol also affects the absorption of calcium. As women are much more susceptible to osteoporosis (brittle bone disease), which is caused by an accelerated loss of calcium from the bones in later life, a regular consumption of alcohol may contribute to the development of the disease as less calcium is laid down in the bones to start with.

BUILDING UP THE BALANCED PLATE

It is no coincidence that the diet that is currently being promoted for better health and reduced risk of long-term disease and premature death from heart disease, stroke and certain forms of cancer forms the foundation

---

The Five Food Groups

Main Food Groups
Cereals and starchy vegetables. These include bread, potatoes, pasta and noodles, rice and breakfast cereals. They also include other cereal grains such as oats, maize, millet and cornmeal and other starchy vegetables like yams and plantains. Beans, peas and lentils can also be included in this group. They provide carbohydrate, dietary fibre, some calcium and iron, B vitamins and are predominantly low in fat. These should form the main part of the diet.
Fruit and vegetables. These include fresh, frozen and canned fruit and vegetables and salad vegetables. Dried fruit and fruit juice can make up some of the choices. They provide vitamins particularly vitamin C, beta-carotene and folic acid, other antioxidants, dietary fibre and some carbohydrate. The darker the vegetables (broccoli, spinach, greens and peppers) the more beta-carotene is present. Beans and peas can be eaten as part of this group. Eat at least five portions per day from this group.
Milk and dairy products. These include milk, cheese, yoghurt and *fromage frais*. This group does not include butter, eggs and cream. These provide protein, calcium, vitamin B$_{12}$, vitamins A and D (lower fat versions contain less of these fat-soluble vitamins). Include two portions per day and choose lower fat versions where possible.
Meat, fish and vegetarian alternatives. These include meat, poultry, fish, eggs, nuts, beans, peas and lentils. This group

includes bacon, salami and meat products such as sausages, beefburgers and pâté. It also includes frozen and canned fish such as fish fingers, fish cakes, tuna and sardines. These provide protein, iron, B vitamins, especially vitamin B$_{12}$, zinc and magnesium. Beans, peas and lentils also provide dietary fibre. Include two portions per day and choose lower fat items where possible.

Non-Main Food Group
Foods containing fat. This includes margarine, butter and other spreading fats (including low fat spreads), cooking oils, oil-based salad dressings, mayonnaise, cream, chocolate, crisps, biscuits, pastries, cakes, puddings, ice cream, rich sauces and gravies. They provide fat, essential fatty acids and some vitamins. Some fat is needed in the diet but high fat foods should be eaten sparingly and where possible lower fat versions should be chosen.
Foods containing sugar. This includes soft drinks, sweets, jam, honey, marmalade, biscuits, pastries, cakes, puddings and ice cream. They provide carbohydrate, some minerals and vitamins and fat in some products (but not others). Should not be included too often or in large amounts. However as energy (and carbohydrate) requirements increase, carbohydrate in the form of sugar-containing food and drinks is invariably needed to top-up intakes to meet requirements (*see* Chapter 4).

---

of the diet for sporting performance. As Chapters 4 and 5 will show, it is only a foundation but it is a good place to start.

A good diet will contain a wide variety of foods in order to ensure that all the nutrients are present in the required amounts. A diet that is restricted to a limited number of foods or to an overall low food intake is unlikely to be meeting all the essential nutritional requirements. This can have implications for the athlete who is constantly required to maintain a low body weight (*see* Chapter 6). There are no 'good' or 'bad' foods. All foods can fit into the overall diet, but the frequency with which some foods appear and infrequency of others will lead to one diet being good while another will be not so good.

Rather than learning how to juggle nutrients, foods can be divided into groups according to the nutrients they provide. By eating the correct proportions of foods from the four main food groups every day and varying the choices within each group as much as possible, it should be possible to enjoy a balanced diet. The size of each portion will

depend on the individual's energy requirement but the actual relative proportions of the groups will be similar.

HEALTHY EATING MESSAGES

It is true that a significant number of the general public would benefit from making some changes to their diet by taking on board the well-publicized healthy eating messages.

Guidelines for a Healthy Diet

Enjoy eating.
Eat a wide variety of different foods.
Eat the right amount to maintain a healthy
 weight.
Eat plenty of foods rich in starch and
 dietary fibre.
Do not eat too much fat.
Do not eat sugary foods too often.
Take care of the vitamins and minerals in
 food.
If drinking alcohol, keep to sensible limits.

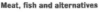

Fruit and vegetables

Bread, other cereals and potatoes

Puffed Wheat

FLAKES

PEA

MILK

MACARONI

BEANS

TUNA

The Balance of Good Health. Reproduced courtesy of the Food Standards Agency.

Meat, fish and alternatives

Foods containing fat
Foods containing sugar

Milk and dairy foods

How appropriate are these guidelines for those who take part in regular exercise?

Certainly, enjoying food and including a wide variety of foods in the daily diet should apply to everybody. Body weight is often an issue for the inactive. Energy requirements are low if little or no physical activity is undertaken and in order to avoid increases in body weight the diet by necessity must be meagre in quantity. However, as physical activity levels rise so does energy requirement with the result that a larger quantity of food can be eaten and enjoyed. However, not all athletes can eat as much as they like. Most athletes find that they perform best at a particular body weight or at least within a narrow range of body weights. For some athletes, however, their sport dictates that they must compete at a particular weight, which is often not their natural weight.

Athletes need to maintain a high carbohydrate intake (*see* Chapter 4) and for many this can only be achieved by eating a variety of foods of both a starchy and sugary nature. Too many starchy foods and foods rich in dietary fibre can make the diet extremely bulky, which can be impractical and not without unwanted side effects. (One of the reasons the general public is being encouraged to increase dietary fibre intake is to help prevent constipation.) The advice to avoid high intakes of fat, take care of vitamins and minerals in food and keep to sensible alcohol limits applies as much to athletes as to the general public.

SOME POPULAR DIETARY MYTHS DEBUNKED

'There are good foods and bad foods.'

All foods provide some nutrients and what matters is to get the balance of foods right. Too much of some foods and not enough of others can result in the wrong proportion of nutrients or the wrong amount of energy being consumed to meet requirements.

'Bread is fattening.'

Bread of any type is low in fat and rich in essential nutrients such as protein, B vitamins and minerals such as iron and calcium. At approximately 80kcal per slice, it is hardly an enemy to those needing to lose weight. It is the high calorie extras that are spread on the bread that can be the real problem.

'Margarine is lower in fat and calories than butter.'

Both butter and margarine contain virtually the same number of calories and total amount of fat. The real difference lies in the type of fat they contain. Low fat spreads contain less total fat and much fewer calories than butter or margarine.

'"No added sugar" means "sugar free".'

'Sugar free' means just that: there is no sugar at all in the product, either present naturally or added by the manufacturer. 'No added sugar' means that no extra sugar has been added by the manufacturer but natural sugars may well be present. For instance, fruit juices may claim to have no added sugar but they still have high natural sugar contents.

'Honey is better than sugar.'

There is no benefit in substituting honey for sugar, apart from the difference in flavour. Sugar and honey are both concentrated sources of carbohydrate (glucose and fructose), with similar glycaemic index factors. Contrary to popular belief, honey contains only negligible amounts of nutrients.

'Extra vitamins will provide more energy.'

Vitamins do not perform magic, they all have particular jobs to do in the body. Only small amounts of vitamins are necessary in the diet for health. It does not follow that having larger amounts will be better for health or energy levels.

'Drinking during meal times hinders digestion.'

Drinking with meals does not dilute digestive juices. Even if it did, this would not affect digestion.

'Drinking milk causes excess mucus production.'

Suggestions that drinking milk increases mucus production and that avoiding milk will alleviate symptoms associated with the common cold have not been backed up by studies. Milk does tend to leave a slightly filmy coating in the mouth or throat due to the creamy texture of the milk but this is not the result of excess mucus production.

'Less food is needed in hot weather than when it is cold.'

The body needs as much energy to sweat and keep cool as it does to keep warm. Although appetite may decrease as the temperature rises, it is important to maintain food intake.

'Brown eggs are healthier than white ones.'

The colour of the shell is completely unrelated to the nutritional content of the egg. In general, a brown hen lays a brown egg and a white hen lays a white egg.

'Low fat milks contain less calcium than whole or full fat milk.'

A pint of semi-skimmed or skimmed milk will actually contain more calcium than a pint of full fat milk. The volume of fat that is skimmed off is replaced with more low fat milk and as calcium is found in this part of the milk, the milk will contain more calcium.

'Eggs are binding.'

Eggs are used to 'bind' ingredients together in cooking but they do not have this effect in the digestive system. They are digested and absorbed in the normal way and therefore cannot be considered a cause of constipation.

CHAPTER 2

Physiology

Several things become apparent as exercise intensity is increased from, for example, standing still to walking, jogging, running and finally going flat out. Heart rate, respiration rate and sweat rate all increase with the increasing work rate. In training, the body is learning to adapt to a given workload so that what was an effort becomes that little bit easier. At subsequent training sessions, a greater workload can be attempted. In other words, sporting performance is being improved. To achieve this a whole spectrum of functions and reactions are changing and adapting at the cellular level.

To look at the physiology and biochemistry of exercise in depth is beyond the scope of this book. However it is important to understand how the diet provides the energy and nutrients needed to support training and competition in all the different situations in which athletes will find themselves. The chains of chemical reactions that take place to make the body function, using food, water and oxygen, are collectively called 'metabolism'.

DIGESTION

How do the meals we eat provide the fuel needed for training and competition?

First the food must be digested and absorbed into the body.

In the Mouth

In the mouth, food is broken down mechanically by chewing. It is mixed with saliva which contains an enzyme (ptyalin) that begins the digestion or breakdown of any carbohydrate that is present. A small amount of fat digestion also begins with the action of the enzyme lipase. Hardly any absorption takes place in the mouth, just a little vitamin C and non-nutrients such as nicotine. The food is then swallowed and reaches the stomach about three seconds later.

In the Stomach

The food is mixed with gastric juice in the stomach and churned up by stomach contractions. Normally about three litres of gastric juice are produced every day. Gastric juice contains the enzyme pepsin which starts the digestion of protein and something called 'intrinsic factor' which is needed for the absorption of vitamin B_{12}. It also contains about 0.2 to 0.4 per cent of hydrochloric acid (much more than is present in acidic food) which destroys most of the bacteria which might be present in food and water. It also makes the stomach conditions acidic so that the pepsin can work effectively. Again, there is a small amount of lipase activity in the stomach.

The stomach is basically a big bag and as such acts as a reservoir for the food. Food usually remains in the stomach for two to four hours

The Digestive System.

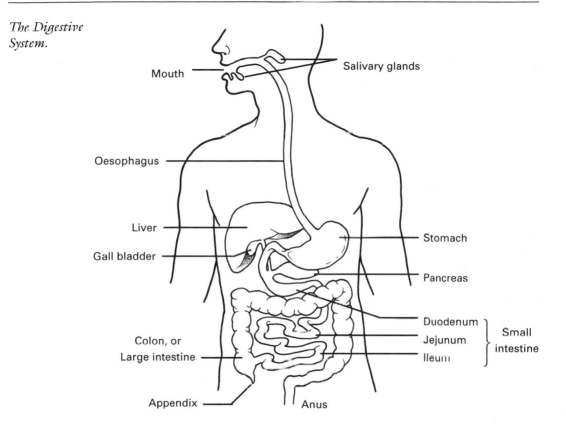

Mouth — Salivary glands

Oesophagus

Liver

Gall bladder

Stomach

Pancreas

Duodenum ⎫
Jejunum ⎬ Small intestine
Ileum ⎭

Colon, or Large intestine

Appendix — Anus

before being passed down the digestive system to the small intestine. Foods rich in carbohydrate pass quickly from the stomach whereas those rich in fat leave more slowly. Tension and nerves, particularly before a competition, can also significantly affect the rate of stomach emptying. Generally, liquids empty from the stomach much faster than solid foods. All these factors must be considered when planning pre-event or pre-match meals (*see* Chapter 5). Again, a small amount of absorption of water, alcohol, sugars and water-soluble vitamins and minerals takes place in the stomach.

In the Small Intestine

The small intestine is somewhat of a misnomer, being the longest part of the digestive system at about three metres in length. Interestingly, after death the loss of tone and elasticity means that it actually *grows* to as much as seven or eight metres long. The small intestine is divided into three distinct sections: the duodenum, the jejunum and lastly the ileum. Most of the digestion and absorption takes place in the small intestine.

The partially digested food is bombarded by digestive juices from three different sources. Bile, which is produced in the liver and stored in the gall bladder, helps to emulsify the fat or break it down into minute droplets so that it can be digested. Juices from the pancreas contain a number of enzymes for breaking down proteins (trypsin and chymotrypsin), fats (lipase) and carbohydrate (amylase) into their simplest forms ready for absorption.

Pancreatic juice is alkaline and neutralizes the acid from the stomach. Finally, the walls of the small intestine contain intestinal juices which in turn contain digestive enzymes so that the final phase of digestion occurs within the intestinal wall.

In the Large Intestine

Once digestion is completed in the small intestine, the remains pass down into the large intestine, another misnomer as it is only about one metre in length. Substances that have not been broken down can be used as a source of nutrients by the colonies of bacteria that are present in the large intestine or colon. Small amounts of B vitamins and vitamin K are manufactured by these bacteria and absorbed into the body. Bacteria present in the large intestine can also produce gas, more commonly referred to as 'wind'.

Absorption

The digestive system is basically a hollow tube with a hole at each end and, until the digested food passes across the gut wall, the gut contents are little more use to the body than the food was while it was still on the plate.

Although a small amount of absorption takes place higher up the digestive system, the small intestine is the main site of absorption for water, alcohol, minerals, vitamins and of course the breakdown products of digestion itself.

Absorption in the small intestine is very efficient. In the clinical situation, patients can have up to half their small intestine removed surgically because of disease without major consequences. The actual surface of the intestine is made up of minute projections which increase the total surface area for absorption up to twenty to forty square metres. Usually at least 95 per cent of the carbohydrate, fat and protein from the digested food is absorbed from the small intestine and eight to nine hours after eating a meal, the fluid residue has passed into the large intestine. Here, as the residue passes slowly down, water is absorbed until finally the waste products or faeces are stored until they are expelled through the anus.

It usually takes one to three days for food to travel from the mouth to the anus. Transit time for men is about fifty-eight hours and for woman about seventy hours. Normal bowel habit is defined by frequency, consistency and amount. Frequency is usually between three

---

Major Enzymes of Digestion

Enzyme	Site of activity	Action
Pytalin	Mouth	Some starch to maltose
Pepsin	Stomach	Protein to peptides
Trypsin	Small intestine	Protein to peptides and amino acids
Chymotrypsin	Small intestine	Protein to peptides and amino acids
Lipase	Small intestine	Fat to fatty acids
Amylase	Small intestine	Starch to maltose
Maltase	Intestinal wall	Maltose to glucose
Sucrase	Intestinal wall	Sucrose to glucose and fructose
Lactase	Intestinal wall	Lactose to glucose and galactose
Peptidases	Intestinal wall	Polypeptides to di-, tri- and oligopeptides and amino acids

times a day and three times a week. In the UK, median stool weight is 106g per day (110g a day for men and 99g a day for women). Such facts can be relevant for the athlete who has to make weight for competition.

What Happens Next?

Once carbohydrate has been broken down into glucose, fructose or galactose, these simple sugars are carried by the blood to the liver where three fates may await them. They may be transported as glucose to all cells of the body to be used directly for energy. Glucose not required for maintenance of normal blood glucose levels may be converted into glycogen and stored in the liver and muscles as a readily available source of energy. Finally these simple sugars may be converted into fatty acids and stored as body fat – another source of energy.

Fatty acids once in the intestinal wall are almost immediately converted back into triglycerides and transported away by the lymphatic system to the blood stream. They are then stored in the body in fat cells which make up the adipose or fatty tissue of the body. Triglycerides are also stored in muscle tissue as small intramuscular fat droplets. There is therefore a large reservoir of fat constantly available as a source of energy.

Peptides entering the intestinal wall are broken down into amino acids and transported straight to the liver. From there they may pass directly into the general circulation and into what is loosely termed the body's pool of amino acids. Here they can be used to build up specific proteins required by the body for growth and repair such as for muscle, hormones, antibodies and so on. Alternatively, some amino acids that are in excess of requirements may be converted into different amino acids. However it is only possible to make non-essential amino acids: the eight essential amino acids that are

required by adults must be supplied by the diet and cannot be made from these excess amino acids.

If there are any excess amino acids, they can in some cases be used for energy. First the amino acid must be deaminated (amino part removed) in the liver, and the remainder converted to urea and excreted by the kidneys. The deaminated part can be used for energy after conversion into glucose or it can be converted and stored as fat.

ENERGY UTILIZATION

Muscle and liver glycogen stores are now topped up, blood glucose levels are steady and there is more potential energy stored in the adipose tissue. How these various energy stores are used during exercise depends on a number of factors including exercise intensity, duration and frequency, diet and fitness level. In sporting performance the aim is to optimize these energy stores and prevent fatigue.

Muscle Fibres

Muscle is made up of distinct muscle fibres, and the speed at which a muscle fibre contracts depends on its ability to convert chemical energy into mechanical energy.

There are three types of skeletal muscle fibres and the type and quantity of each muscle fibre type is genetically determined. However the characteristics of the fibres can be changed substantially by following appropriate training programmes. Increases in muscle size as a result of training are due to an increase in the size of the fibres already present rather than to an increase in the number of fibres. The greater the number and size of fibres, the greater the strength of the muscle. (Some increase in strength is also due to the central nervous system being able to develop the

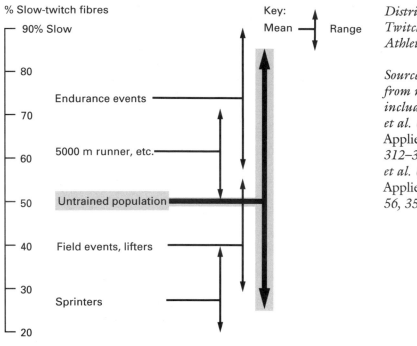

% Slow-twitch fibres

Key: Mean —|— Range

Distribution of Slow Twitch Fibres in Different Athletes.

Source: Summary of data from many sources, including Gollnick, P.D. et al. (1972). Journal of Applied Physiology, 33, *312–319 and Tesch, P. et al. (1984).* Journal of Applied Physiology, *56, 35–38).*

capacity to recruit more motor units for contraction.)

Energy Systems

There are three distinct energy systems and which one is used will determine how quickly energy is produced and therefore the exercise intensity level that can be achieved. Each muscle fibre possesses all three systems but the dominance of one energy system over another gives the fibre its own energy characteristics.

The end point of each system is the same, namely the production of an energy-rich compound called adenosine triphosphate or ATP, often referred to as the body's 'universal energy currency'. ATP is used for all energy requiring processes in cells. It is broken down in the cell and the chemical energy released is made available for muscle contraction.

Without ATP muscles cannot contract and no work can be accomplished.

Unfortunately, muscle only contains a very small amount of ATP, just enough to exercise maximally for one second. To maintain muscle contractions and therefore the ability to carry on exercising, ATP has to be continually resynthesized from adenosine diphosphate (ADP), also present in muscles. The more intense the level of exercise, the more rapidly this resynthesis must take place. The three energy systems allow the body to cope with the various demands placed on exercising muscles.

Phosphocreatine System

The phosphocreatine system uses another energy-rich compound, creatine phosphate (CP) as well as ATP. CP breaks down in a similar way to ATP to release energy very

---

Characteristics of Muscle Fibre Types

Type I (slow twitch or slow oxidative fibres)
- Contract and relax slowly (but still many times a second).
- Resistant to fatigue.
- Important for aerobic endurance exercise.
- Elite marathon runners will have a high proportion of Type I fibres.

Type IIa (fast twitch or fast oxidative fibres)
- Can work both aerobically and anaerobically (with or without oxygen).
- Less aerobic capacity than slow twitch fibres.

- More aerobic capacity than fast glycolytic fibres.
- Moderate fatigue resistance.
- Fibres seem to change their characteristics in response to training loads or stresses.

Type IIb (fast twitch or fast glycolytic fibres)
- Contract twice as fast as slow twitch fibres.
- Fatigue quickly.
- Important for anaerobic exercise.
- Elite sprinters will have a high proportion of Type IIb fibres.

---

rapidly but the muscle cannot use this energy directly for muscle contraction. Instead, it is used to resynthesize the ATP. CP is also limited in the muscle and probably only supplies enough energy for a further five to ten seconds.

The ATP-CP energy system is a characteristic of the fast-twitch fibres (Type IIa and Type IIb). This energy system does not need oxygen and is often referred to as an anaerobic energy source. It is capable of producing energy very quickly but only for short periods of time. Well-planned training programmes can help to improve the concentration of CP in muscles. More recently, researchers have been investigating the use of creatine supplementation to boost the whole body creatine pool (*see* Chapter 7).

This energy system is used for fast bursts of exercise such as a throw, jump, lift or a short 20-metre sprint.

Glycolysis

The glycolytic system primarily uses carbohydrate as its fuel, most of which is obtained from the glycogen stored in the muscles. The breakdown of muscle glycogen is called glycogenolysis and it leads to a process called glycolysis in which ATP can be produced rapidly, although not as rapidly as in the ATP-CP system.

Glycolysis occurs in both the presence and absence of oxygen. At rest, the requirement for ATP is low and the required rate of glycolysis can be sustained by oxygen obtained by normal breathing patterns. As exercise intensity level increases, so the rate of glycolysis must increase if the demand for ATP is to be met. Eventually the requirement for ATP can no longer be met by aerobic glycolysis and proportionally more anaerobic glycolysis is needed to meet the ATP need. This process results in a much faster production of ATP.

However, the glucose (from glycogen) is only partially broken down and by a series of chemical reactions it is converted into lactic acid with the production of hydrogen ions. As acid conditions begin to build up, the functioning of the body becomes impaired and the muscles fatigue very quickly. The pain felt in the legs and arms after a few minutes of intense exercise is due to this process. It is the resulting hydrogen ion and its effect on pH, rather than the lactate anion, which is considered to be detrimental to muscle function.

The increasing acidity reduces the activity of a key glycolytic enzyme so the glycolysis is inhibited. The more acid conditions also impair muscle contraction. In addition, the fall in pH may have a negative effect on feelings of well being and other psychological parameters. Research suggests that the use of alkaline salts such as sodium bicarbonate may help to neutralize the hydrogen ion, thus reducing the acidity and delaying the onset of fatigue. Lactic acid can be used as an energy source but it tends to be produced faster than the muscles can use it. The end result is therefore still the same: an eventual accumulation of lactic acid in muscles.

This energy system is capable of producing energy at a fairly rapid rate but it cannot produce energy for prolonged periods. It is the preferred energy system used, for example, in 400 or 800-metre sprints, weight training sessions or any all-out 90-second activity.

Oxygen System

The oxygen energy system can use a variety of fuels to produce ATP but its primary fuel sources are carbohydrate and fat and, as its name implies, it also requires oxygen. This system is often referred to as the 'aerobic energy system'.

The main source of carbohydrate is glucose which is stored in limited amounts in the muscles as glycogen. More glucose is stored in the liver as glycogen and this can be released into the blood stream and transported to the muscles, but again the liver stores are limited. The main source of fat for muscular energy during exercise is free fatty acids (FFA). Some fats (triglycerides) are stored in small amounts actually within the muscle and these can be broken down into FFA to be taken up by the oxygen energy system. However the bulk of body fat is stored under the skin and in deposits deeper in the body (adipose tissue). Even in the leanest of sportsmen and women, this store represents a vast potential of energy. Protein is not normally used for energy production but under some conditions, for instance during endurance events, it can be a source of energy for the oxygen system.

The oxygen system produces greater quantities of ATP than the other systems but at a slower rate. How slowly depends on the fuel that is used. For a given amount of oxygen, more energy can be produced by metabolizing carbohydrate than fat. Carbohydrate is therefore a more efficient fuel but its limited storage capacity can have a limiting effect on performance. As glycogen stores are used up, the rate of glycolysis and therefore glucose oxidation decreases progressively. The rate of ATP production slows, the power output decreases and the athlete slows down. This is commonly known as 'hitting the wall' in running and (rather unfortunately) 'bonking' in cycling. Slowing down allows the slower fatty acid oxidation to provide a greater proportion of the energy demand.

Energy Stores in the Body		
	Male	*Female*
Liver glycogen	90g	70g
Muscle glycogen	400g	300g
Intramuscular fat	500g	500g
Adipose tissue	7–10kg	12–20kg

Normal body stores of fat and carbohydrate in a typical 70kg male athlete and a typical 60kg female athlete.

Uses of Energy Sources in Exercise

At rest, about two thirds of the body's energy requirements are derived from fat metabolism and a third from the metabolism of carbohydrate. During exercise, the relative amounts of fat and carbohydrate used will depend on the intensity, duration and frequency of exercise as well as the diet that has been regularly consumed (as this will have influenced fuel stores) and the fitness level of the individual.

Amino acids are not a major energy source during exercise. Proteins have a unique function (growth and repair) and supplies must be preserved for this use rather than wasting them on energy production, which is the main function of carbohydrate and fat. When carbohydrate intake is very low, protein can be utilized for energy production. However, as it is an aerobic source of fuel, it can only be used in low to moderate intensity exercise.

Fatty acids, another aerobic source of energy, cannot be utilized in high intensity exercise. However this is a vital energy source for endurance exercise as it provides a virtually unlimited supply, even in the leanest of athletes. Training can help to increase the body's capacity for oxygen uptake and therefore increase the body's ability to use fat as an energy source.

Carbohydrate in the form of muscle glycogen is the body's immediate energy source. It can be called on at the onset of exercise as well as during high intensity exercise. For a given volume of oxygen, carbohydrate produces 12 per cent more energy than fat. Endurance training can increase the capacity of muscles to store glycogen. Trained athletes have 20 to 50 per cent more muscle glycogen than untrained people do. A trained endurance runner will therefore be more effective at carbohydrate loading prior to a marathon than a less well-trained runner (*see* Chapter 5).

Diet

The relative contributions of carbohydrate and fat in the diet will affect how much glycogen and fat is available as an energy source during exercise. Storage of muscle glycogen is limited, unlike fat storage which is unlimited, and a poor carbohydrate intake will result in even lower muscle glycogen stores. This will result in an inability to sustain high intensity levels of exercise.

Fitness

Fitness level can be improved by training. Appropriate training will result in an increased ability of the muscles to use fat as a source of fuel in aerobic exercise, therefore sparing the limited supplies of carbohydrate. It will also give an increased ability to store muscle glycogen. In addition, the build up of lactic acid will begin at a higher aerobic intensity.

Which Energy System for Which Sport?

At the start of exercise, the anaerobic pathway is the main energy source as it takes time for the heart and circulation to transport oxygen to the muscles and for the muscles to then utilize it. This highlights the importance of the warm-up, which acts almost like an alert for the body to prepare for action. If the exercise is of a high intensity nature, the anaerobic system will continue to supply the required energy. For moderate to low intensity exercise, the aerobic pathway will kick in to supply the required energy. In reality it is not just a matter of switching from one system to another but of the systems being used together, with the relevant pathways and metabolic reactions being phased in and out.

At one end of the scale, sprinting can be classified as an anaerobic exercise and, at the other end, marathon running can be classified as an aerobic exercise. However the vast majority of sports utilize both the anaerobic and aerobic systems. Even the marathon runner will use the anaerobic system more at the start of the race, when tackling a hilly course, or when attempting a sprint finish. Team sports tend to be a combination of short, high intensity bursts with periods of lower intensity exercise in between.

The 800-metre race is an excellent example of how the two anaerobic systems together with the aerobic system are all utilized. At the start of the race, the ATP-CP system will provide the fuel for the first seconds. Anaerobic glycolysis will be the main fuel for the first 100 to 400 metres, the fastest part of the race when oxygen demand is greater than the body can supply. By the time the bell goes for the last lap, the respiratory and circulatory systems will have adjusted to the increased demands on them and the aerobic system begins to kick in. The final 200 metres, the dash for the line, again demands more oxygen than the body can supply and the anaerobic glycolysis comes up with the goods, but at the price of accumulated lactate and hydrogen ions. This highlights the importance of active recovery and the warm-down period to restore all systems back to normal resting states, including the conversion of lactate into less toxic substances which can then be removed by the circulating blood.

FLUID BALANCE

Fluid loss during exercise is linked to the need to maintain the body temperature between narrow limits. A wide variation in skin temperature can be tolerated but the deep structures of the body must be maintained around 37°C. The body is somewhat inefficient at converting the energy it gets from foods into useful work and much of the available energy is lost as heat in the process. During exercise the demand for energy is increased and the rate of heat production rises correspondingly.

At rest the rate of heat production is about 1kcal per minute. However, a well-trained athlete may be producing heat at a rate of 20kcal per minute throughout a two or three hour training session or competition – a huge amount of heat which must be removed from the body. However the increased heat production soon overloads the usual mechanisms of heat loss (conduction, convection and radiation). The body must now turn to another method of heat loss, namely the evaporation of sweat which is secreted onto the skin surface. Evaporation of one litre of water from the skin removes 590kcal of heat from the body. High rates of sweat loss are therefore essential during prolonged intense exercise if the rise in body temperature is to be limited and the loss of performance capacity that would otherwise occur is to be minimized.

The downside of the process is that the loss of large amounts of sweat can lead to dehydration and electrolyte losses which will also have a negative effect on performance. The rate of sweating is highly variable and individual losses exceeding two litres per hour can occur in certain circumstances.

What Happens When the Body Becomes Dehydrated?

If fluid is not replaced and the body becomes dehydrated, not only is performance impaired but also health is put at risk. The plasma volume (the fluid component of blood) is needed to take oxygen and fuel to the working muscles, remove waste products and carry heat to the skin for removal. If sweat losses are not replaced the plasma volume drops. This causes the heart rate to increase in order to keep up the cardiac output (the amount of blood pumped out each beat). Blood flow to the exercising muscles takes priority so blood flow to the skin is reduced, sweat rate drops and body temperature rises. This affects performance but if unchecked when exercising in the heat, it can lead to heat exhaustion. A loss of body water corresponding to 2 per cent body weight will start to impair performance and losses in excess of 5 per cent body weight can decrease work capacity by as much as 30 per cent. Heat illness can occur when 5 to 6 per cent of body weight is lost.

Rate of Sweating

Individuals sweat at different rates, even in the same conditions. The rate of sweating depends on a number of factors.

Exercise intensity. The rate of heat production and therefore sweat production is dependent on the exercise intensity and duration. The harder the exercise, the greater the heat production and therefore sweat production. In duration events, the intensity will be less but the time spent exercising will be greater so total sweat losses can be considerable.

Environmental temperature. As the temperature of the surroundings increases, the effectiveness of heat loss by conduction, convection and radiation decreases. Indeed when ambient temperature exceeds body temperature, heat is actually gained from the environment so that the body has to rely on evaporation of sweat to cool the body down. As the temperature increases further the amount of evaporation required to maintain the body temperature increases and consequently the amount of fluid lost increases as well.

Humidity. If the surrounding air is very dry most if not all of the sweat produced will be evaporated. However very humid air already contains a lot of moisture, up to the point

where it cannot take up more. Even though large quantities of sweat 'bead' on the skin, they eventually just roll off rather than evaporating. As it is the process of evaporation that cools the body down, not just the production of sweat, this will contribute little to the cooling down process. There will therefore be fluid losses without the benefit of temperature regulation. Evaporative cooling is also restricted by continually drying the skin with a towel before the sweat has had a chance to evaporate. An element of wind speed will help evaporation – an advantage that cyclists may have over other sports.

Body surface area. Compared to men, women have a relatively large surface area to weight ratio. In other words, per unit of body weight the female has a larger surface exposed to the environment. Consequently under identical conditions of heat exposure, women will tend to cool at a faster rate than men do. Women are also believed to sweat more economically than men do.

Hydration status. If dehydration is allowed to continue unchecked, sweat production and skin blood flow may become limited which in turn will lead to less fluid becoming available at the skin for evaporation and a reduction in body cooling. In other words, the more dehydrated an athlete becomes, the slower the rate of sweating and the greater the likelihood of a rise in body temperature and the subsequent problems that can bring.

Acclimatization. A training session well tolerated in cool conditions may become extremely taxing if undertaken on an unusually hot day. However repeated exposure to exercise in a hot environment results in improved capacity for exercise and less discomfort on exposure to heat. The physiological adaptive changes that improve heat tolerance are collectively termed 'heat acclimatization'. The major acclimatization occurs during the first

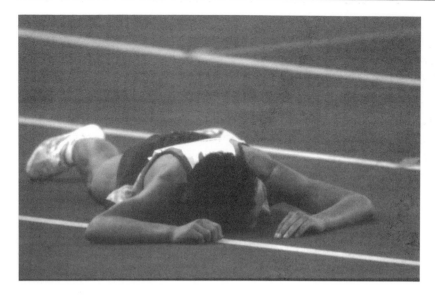

Young Cho Hwang Kor after winning the Marathon Gold at the Barcelona Olympic Games in 1992.

week of heat exposure and is essentially complete by the end of ten days.

Clothing. Heat loss by sweat evaporation may become severely restricted by inappropriate clothing. Multiple layers of clothing, nylon training suits or any other sports protective clothing may almost totally block sweat evaporation. Heat loss by convection and radiation will also be cut back considerably so total heat loss could be reduced to potentially critical levels.

FATIGUE

The onset of fatigue results in loss of performance so athletes will want to avoid, at least for as long as possible, the point at which fatigue sets in. The causes of fatigue are many and sports scientists continue to look for ways to help athletes beat fatigue. The use of creatine and buffering agents such as sodium bicarbonate are both examples of how science has helped to combat fatigue.

Diet has an enormous role to play in fatigue prevention. If an athlete follows the correct diet and fluid strategies and achieves his or her optimum body composition, the onset of fatigue can be delayed.

GLOSSARY OF TERMS

Acclimatization. This is the process of adaptation to repeated bouts of exercise in hot climates which results in improvement in exercise time to fatigue.

Acclimation. This is the same process as for acclimatization except that the adaptation takes place in controlled laboratory settings.

Acid. A chemical which splits up in solution to yield hydrogen ions (H+). Acids have a pH of less than 7 and are neutralized by alkalis.

Alkali. A chemical that mops up H+ and therefore neutralizes acids. Alkalis have a pH greater than 7.

Buffer. A buffer is a substance that helps to prevent changes in pH.

VO2max. VO2max or maximum oxygen consumption is the maximum amount of oxygen that an individual can use in one minute. It is a measure of an individual's aerobic capacity.

pH. Acidity or alkalinity is measured on the pH scale. pH 7 is neutral; a pH value of less than 7 is progressively more acidic; a pH value of more than 7 is progressively more alkaline.

Power. The rate of doing work or the rate of energy transfer.

Strength. The force that a muscle can exert in one maximal effort.

Work. The application of a force through a distance.

Work rate. Work performed per unit time, or in other words, power.

CHAPTER 3

Body Composition

Actual body weight will be of great importance to those athletes who compete in weight category sports, but it is the make up or composition of the body, rather than body weight itself, which will be important to most athletes. Excess body fat may not be a disadvantage to an archer or pistol shooter but in other sports excess body fat can reduce speed, strength and endurance. Consider two athletes weighing exactly the same but with different body compositions who compete against each other. The person with a higher percentage of muscle and lower percentage of body fat than the other will have the advantage. There are very few sports where fat could be considered an advantage, apart from sumo wrestling and long distance swimming where the extra body fat provides insulation and additional buoyancy. Equally, body fat which is too low is not only counterproductive to performance but also dangerous to health and fitness.

Although the body is made up of many different types of tissues, muscle and fat cause the greatest variations in total body weight. Increases in blood volume with increased fitness can account for weight increases of up to 1kg and bone mass may also increase with exercise (although bone mass tends to decrease with age from about thirty-five years old). The amount of body fat is measured by assessing the fat-free mass and fat mass of an individual. The fat-free mass, sometimes referred to as 'lean mass' includes water, muscle, bone, connective tissues and internal organs. The fat mass includes adipose tissue and fat present in other tissues.

BODY FAT

Body fat is made up of essential fat and storage fat. Essential fat is found in the brain, nerves, bone marrow, heart tissue and cell walls. About 10 per cent of the body weight of women and about 3 per cent of the body weight of men is accounted for by essential fat. The higher percentage of essential fat in women is due to essential fat associated with the pelvic and breast region, which is known as 'gender-specific fat' and plays a key role in reproduction.

Reducing the percentage of body fat towards that of essential body fat alone will impair physiological function and the capacity of the body to exercise. It will also carry certain health risks. It is generally accepted that the minimal body fat level for men should not be less than 5 per cent. There is no consensus on the minimal fat per cent for women though ranges from 12 to 16 per cent body fat have been quoted. The essential fat percentage is definitely not the optimal fat percentage.

Storage fat (adipose tissue) is a major source of fuel. The fat is stored in fat cells (adipocytes). Each fat cell contains about 45µg of fat with a capacity to gain up to twice this amount. Women have considerably more

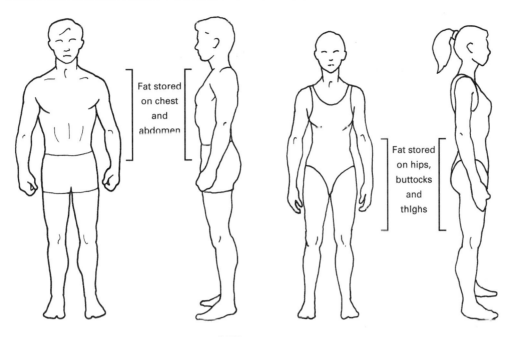

Relative Fat Distribution in Men and Women.

storage fat than men do. Again, the reasons for this are tied up with reproduction, the difference in absolute terms being similar to the energy cost of pregnancy.

Storage fat is found under the skin (subcutaneous fat) and around the vital organs where it has a protective function. When overweight and obese people lose weight, the amount of fat in the adipocytes drops but the actual number of adipocytes does not change.

MEASURING BODY WEIGHT AND BODY COMPOSITION

Body Weight

The simplest method of determining your body weight is to carry out regular weighing, perhaps weekly. This must be carried out under the same conditions (no shoes, minimal or no clothing, at the same time of day, using the same set of scales, in the same nourished and hydrated state and after a successful visit to the lavatory). The preferred and most convenient time is often immediately after getting out of bed in the morning.

Weight may fluctuate by up to 2kg or more on a daily basis, particularly for women, so it is important not to get obsessed with the precise readings but to use them as an indication of the general trend in body weight. Comparing height and weight with standard height and weight charts can also be misleading. These charts are normally based on the average weight of a sample population group (usually those seeking life insurance) and are not necessarily representative. Most athletes have a higher percentage of muscle than the general population, and muscle is much denser than fat. In other words, a kilogram of fat takes up more space than a kilogram of muscle. Using standard tables could lead to the conclusion that athletes are overweight when they are actually probably

47

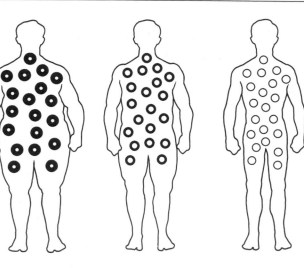

*Fat Cell Changes
Associated with
Weight Reduction.*

Body mass	149 kg	103 kg	75 kg
Fat cell size	0.9 μg per cell	0.6 μg per cell	0.2 μg per cell
Fat cell number	75 billion	75 billion	75 billion

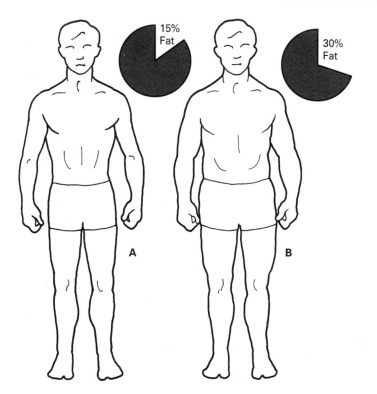

*Possible Variation
in Body
Composition for the
Same Weight.*

underfat looking leaner but weighing more. The *excess* weight is a reflection of the increased muscle mass resulting from a well-structured training programme, not an indication of a dietary over-indulgence. Scales are biased towards tall, thin people and do no favours for short, muscular people.

Body Mass Index

There is no ideal weight for all people of the same height so reference to a range of values is more realistic. The body mass index (BMI), based on the relationship between height and weight provides this range. However, it still does not take into account body composition. An athlete with a high percentage of muscle but low body fat percentage could have a BMI which classifies them as overweight whereas a sedentary individual with more fat and less muscle could have a BMI which puts him or her firmly in the 'normal' category.

Calculating and Interpreting Body Mass Index (BMI)

Body mass index = $\dfrac{\text{weight}}{(\text{height})^2}$
(BMI)

(Weight measured in kilograms and height in metres.)

For example, a male weighing 73kg and 1.85m tall would have a BMI of 21.3, which is within the normal range.

$$BMI = \frac{73}{(1.85)^2} = 21.3$$

Classification	BMI
Underweight	< 18.5
Normal	18.5–24.9
Overweight	25–29.9
Obese class I	30–34.9
Obese class II	35–39.9
Obese class III	> 40

Body Composition

Measurement of body composition can be helpful in a variety of ways, particularly for monitoring desired changes, identifying health risks of athletes with very low body fat levels and estimating ideal and minimal body weights. For instance an athlete competing in a weight category sport may need to know if it is feasible to drop a weight category.

There are a variety of methods available for measuring body composition, which can be divided into reference body composition methods and field techniques. Reference body composition measurements (densitometry, often referred to as the 'gold standard', isotope dilution methods, dual energy X-ray absorptiometry, computerized tomographic scanning and magnetic resonance imaging) are beyond the scope of this book. Field techniques (the more practical methods that are used in gyms and training venues) include measurements of skinfold thickness, bio-electrical impedance analysis (BIA) and near-infrared interactance (NIRI).

Skinfold Thicknesses

This method involves the measurement of a fold of subcutaneous fat at one or more sites which is then interpreted using equations to estimate fat mass. In the UK the equations of Durnin and Womersley are the most widely used for adults. They are based on skin-fold measurements at four sites: triceps, biceps, subscapular and supra-iliac. Measurements are made using calipers which exert a standardized pressure on the site that is being measured.

Skinfold tests are probably the most widely used technique for estimating fat mass. The advantage of this method is that it is non-invasive (although depending on which sites are used some degree of undressing may be

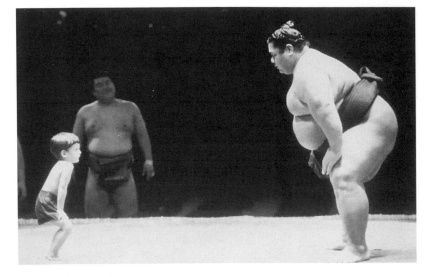

Sumo wrestling.

necessary), costs little once the calipers have been acquired and can be used to highlight fat distribution (different parts of the body). The disadvantages of the method are that it is affected by the skill of the technician, the type of calipers used, the ease or otherwise of measuring the individual (obese individuals are definitely not easy to measure) and the prediction equations that are used to calculate the fat mass.

Bioelectrical Impedance Analysis (BIA)

This method is based on passing a small current of electricity between electrodes placed on the hands and feet. The voltage drop is measured to give an estimate of the body resistance or 'impedance'. The current is passed through the water and electrolyte component of lean tissue. The electrical resistance is proportional to the body water volume, which is then used to estimate lean body mass. Fat mass is then calculated by subtracting lean body mass from body weight.

The advantages of this method are that it is rapid, non-invasive and non-intrusive, relatively inexpensive and does not require any particular degree of technical skill. On the downside, the results are affected by the state of the athlete at the time of measurement. For the most accurate results the athlete should not have eaten or drunk anything for four hours, not exercised during the last twelve hours, not drunk alcohol within the last forty-eight hours, not used diuretics within the last seven days and must have urinated within the last thirty minutes. If these precautions are not taken each time an athlete is measured, results could very well be misleading.

Near-Infrared Interactance (NIRI)

This is a relatively new technique which involves irradiating tissues with a beam of near-infrared radiation. The measured optical density of the reflected radiation is influenced by the composition of the tissues through which the light is passing. This method is still in experimental stages. Prediction equations are used to interpret measurements over only one site and attempts to make measurements over multiple sites have so far proved unsuccessful. A large proportion of variation occurs because weight, height, age, sex and activity are all included in the prediction

SPORT	MEN	WOMEN
Baseball, softball	8–14	12–18
Basketball	6–12	10–16
Body building	5–8	6–12
Canoeing and kayaking	6–12	10–16
Cycling	5–11	8–15
Fencing	8–12	10–16
Football	6–18	—
Golf	10–16	12–20
Gymnastics	5–12	8–16
Horse racing	6–12	10–16
Ice and field hockey	8–16	12–18
Orienteering	5–12	8–16
Pentathlon	—	8–15
Racketball	6–14	10–18
Rowing	6–14	8–16
Rugby	6–16	—
Skating	5–12	8–16
Skiing	7–15	10–18
Ski jumping	7–15	10–18
Soccer	6–14	10–18
Swimming	6–12	10–18
Synchronized swimming	—	10–18
Tennis	6–14	10–20
Track and field		
Running events	5–12	8–15
Field events	8–18	12–20
Triathlon	5–12	8–15
Volleyball	7–15	10–18
Weight lifting	5–12	10–18
Wrestling	5–16	—

Relative Body Fat Ranges for Different Sports. Adapted from J.H. Wilmore and D.L. Costill, Physiology of Sport and Exercise *(Champaign; IL: Human Kinetics, 1994).*

equation for calculating body fat. However, the measurement is simple and non-invasive and the cost of carrying out the test is very low once the equipment has been purchased.

Not everyone has access to reliable scales, let alone skinfold calipers or other methods of assessing body composition. For many people, the eye (or clothing) can be an acceptable rough method of assessing body composition. However some people do have distorted body images of themselves, believing that they are overweight or fat, when actually they are unhealthily thin.

If body fat measurements are taken, it is important that athletes understand the limitations of such measurements. They are most useful when assessed alongside other fitness tests so that a complete picture of the athlete's overall profile can be determined. The most important factor will be how well the athlete is performing. It is pointless battling to reach a lower body fat measurement if speed, strength and stamina are dipping. Every person has his or her own ideal weight and body composition and setting body fat targets for whole squads or teams can be counter-productive. The data (on left) shows how much variation in body fat measurements there can be, not only between athletes taking part in different sports but also between athletes competing within the same sport.

CHAPTER 4

The Training Diet

Many people believe that the competition diet is crucial (and certainly getting it wrong on the day of competition can have disastrous consequences). However, it is the day-to-day diet that supports the training programme and this is where nutrition can have its greatest impact.

The primary dietary requirement for an athlete in training is to consume a well-balanced, nutritionally complete diet that will meet the additional nutrient and fluid demands imposed by the training load. In other words it must be a healthy diet, that allows the athlete to train hard, to recover from each training session and maintain his or her own *ideal* body weight (unless there is a need to reduce weight for competition).

Training brings about adaptations which enable athletes to improve their performance by training and competing at higher exercise intensities or as the Olympic motto *Citius, Altius, Fortius* translates 'swifter, higher, stronger'. To train regularly and intensively, the athlete must have recovered from the previous training session and a number of body systems need to have been restored to normal. The return to normal of these systems is invariably helped by what and when an athlete eats and drinks after exercise. For example, replenishment of the body's glycogen stores is essential for successful recovery from exercise and to prepare the body for the next training session.

ESTABLISHING ENERGY REQUIREMENTS

How much energy an athlete needs and therefore how much the athlete needs to eat and drink depends on that individual's basal metabolic rate (BMR) and daily physical activity level. Athletes often want to know what their energy intake should be (as indeed they want to know what their ideal body weight should be) and therefore how much they should be eating. As discussed later in this chapter, the quality or make-up of the diet is as important as quantity. However in some situations, relying on perceived energy levels and an acceptable body weight and composition may not be enough and an estimate of energy requirements is required.

Energy expenditure (EE) is the sum of the basal metabolic rate (BMR) plus the cost of all the day's activities. The contribution to total daily energy expenditure of the thermic effect of food (TEF) and adaptive thermogenesis (AT) are small in comparison and are not normally taken into account in the calculation of energy expenditure.

There are two methods that can be used to calculate energy requirements, one slightly more complicated than the other, but as a result more accurate.

Physical Activity Level (PAL)

The first method of calculating energy requirements is based on the Physical Activity

Calculated Physical Activity Level (PAL) of Adults at Three Levels Each of Occupational and Non-occupational Activity

Non-occupational Activity			*Occupational Activity*				
	Light		Moderate		Moderate/Heavy	
	Male	Female	Male	Female	Male	Female
Non-active	1.4	1.4	1.6	1.5	1.7	1.5
Moderately active	1.5	1.5	1.7	1.6	1.8	1.6
Very active	1.6	1.6	1.8	1.7	1.9	1.7

Level (PAL) and requires the athlete to make an assumption of the energy demands of both his or her occupation or job and the remainder of a normal day. The BMR must be calculated (*see* Chapter 1) and then using the appropriate PAL, the energy expenditure and therefore energy requirement can be calculated.

Physical Activity Ratio (PAR)

The second method for calculating energy requirements is based on the Physical Activity Ratio (PAR) for each activity of the day. This requires the athlete to keep an activity diary.

An Example of Calculating EE Using the PAL Method

Assumptions: male athlete, 23 years old, weighing 70kg has light job and a moderately active lifestyle out of working hours.

$BMR = (15.1 \times 70) + 692 = 1{,}749$
$PAL = 1.5$
$EE = BMR \times PAL = 1{,}749 \times 1.5 = 2{,}624\text{kcal}$

Each activity can then be assigned the appropriate PAR and, together with the calculated BMR, the energy expenditure can be calculated.

PAR for Various Activities

PAR 1.2 (1.0 to 1.4)
Lying at rest: reading
Sitting at rest: watching TV, writing, listening to the radio, eating
Standing at rest

PAR 1.6 (1.5 to 1.8)
Sitting: driving
Standing: washing up, ironing, general office work

PAR 2.1 (1.9 to 2.4)
Standing: cleaning, cooking, playing snooker

PAR 2.8 (2.5 to 3.3)
Standing: dressing and undressing,

showering, making beds
Walking: 3 to 4km per hour

PAR 3.7 (3.4 to 4.4)
Standing: gardening
Walking: 4 to 6km per hour; playing golf

PAR 4.8 (4.5 to 5.9)
Walking: 6 to 7km per hour
Exercise: dancing, moderate swimming, gently cycling, slow jogging

PAR 6.9 (6.0 to 7.9)
Walking: uphill with a load or cross-country, climbing stairs
Exercise: average jogging, cycling
Sport: football, swimming, tennis, skiing

An Example of Calculating EE Using the PAR Method

Assumptions: male athlete, 23 years old, weight 70kg.
BMR = $(15.1 \times 70) + 692 = 1,749$

Activity	Hours	PAR	Total Energy Cost in kcal (BMR × PAR × Time/24)
Sleeping	8	1	583
Showering and dressing	0.5	2.8	102
Sitting eating breakfast and reading paper	0.5	1.2	44
Driving to work	1	1.6	117
Sitting at work (and eating lunch)	8	1.2	700
Driving to training	1	1.6	117
Training (hard session)	1.5	6.9	754
Showering and dressing	0.5	1.2	44
Meal out (sitting)	1	1.2	88
Watching TV	2	1.2	175

Total energy expenditure over the 24-hour period = 2,724kcal

This example shows how energy requirements are primarily determined by training load (intensity, frequency and duration), type of employment (if applicable) and body weight (because of the bearing on basal metabolic rate). For example, the likely energy requirements for a heavyweight Olympic rower with a body weight of 100kg doing two or three training sessions a day will obviously be great. Such an energy expenditure may exceed the nutritional intake of a normal eating pattern and explains why many athletes find they need to supplement their meals with regular snacks of a suitable nature between meals.

CARBOHYDRATE: THE UNIVERSAL FUEL SOURCE

The most important nutrient for sporting performance is carbohydrate, which is the primary fuel for muscle contraction as much for the endurance athlete as for the athlete competing on strength and speed. Unfortunately, the body is only able to store a limited amount of carbohydrate. Total energy turnover and the proportion of the energy demand met by carbohydrate breakdown increases as the exercise intensity increases. Thus athletes participating in explosive sports such as sprinting or during weight training sessions will rely almost exclusively on carbohydrate for their fuel source.

Muscle glycogen can also become depleted after only fifteen to thirty minutes of exercise performed at very high intensities (90 to 130 per cent VO2max) in intervals of one to five minutes of exercise with rest periods in between each exercise bout.

Although fat can provide fuel at low intensities, it cannot support exercise above 60 to 65 per cent of maximal oxygen uptake (VO2max).

Intense training loads undertaken by competitive athletes thus place large demands on their carbohydrate reserves. Not only

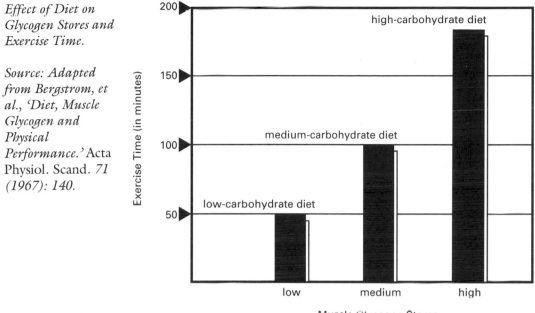

Effect of Diet on Glycogen Stores and Exercise Time.

Source: Adapted from Bergstrom, et al., 'Diet, Muscle Glycogen and Physical Performance.' Acta Physiol. Scand. *71 (1967): 140.*

exercise intensity but also the duration of exercise affects the glycogen stores. After two to three hours of continuous exercise at 60 to 80 per cent VO2max, muscle glycogen becomes depleted and the athlete fatigues. In team sports such as football, rugby and hockey involving high intensity intermittent exercise, a heavy demand is also placed on the body's stores of glycogen.

Chronic glycogen depletion may cause chronic fatigue in its own right, thus reducing the ability to recover from and respond to a heavy training programme (*see* Chapter 12). With daily training sessions and in some cases two or even more sessions in the same day, athletes have to recover over hours rather than days. Restocking both muscle and liver glycogen stores is essential but this can only be achieved in the short time available if athletes eat carbohydrate-rich diets.

Athletes undertaking high intensity training need to consume at least 60 per cent of their total energy intake as carbohydrate.

Unfortunately though many athletes recognize the importance of consuming a high carbohydrate diet, their diet often contains no more carbohydrate than the 40 to 45 per cent of total energy intake of the general public. On this low intake athletes can expect to experience chronic fatigue, particularly during periods of intense training. It is only by having a high carbohydrate intake on a regular basis, thus making sure that each training session is started with muscles well stocked with glycogen, that the onset of fatigue can be avoided or at least delayed.

Symptoms of Fatigue

An increase in training load can cause temporary feelings of tiredness but these soon disappear as the athlete adapts to the greater workload. Tiredness may also be due to lack of sleep and poor recovery time between training sessions. However, if poor nutrition is the cause of the tiredness, simple changes in

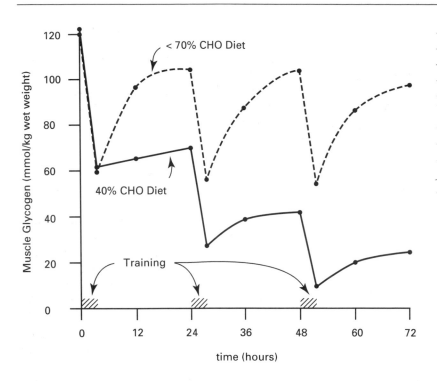

Replacement of Muscle Glycogen After Prolonged Daily Training Sessions.

Source: D.L. Costill and J.M. Miller, International Journal of Sports Medicine, 1: 2–14 (1980).

eating habits may rectify the problem. Symptoms of fatigue caused by a low carbohydrate intake include muscle heaviness, poor energy levels in training, a feeling of great effort but without the expected outcome, and progressive tiredness over the training week. Athletes who have to restrict their energy intake in order to maintain a low body weight (for example gymnasts, lightweight rowers, boxers and wrestlers) are often constantly fatigued because the energy restriction leads to a permanently low carbohydrate intake.

Carbohydrate Intake on a Weight Basis

Though the carbohydrate requirement is frequently cited as a percentage of total energy, a requirement related to body weight is far more practical and takes into account not only the different intakes of men and women but also the different levels of training intensity.

Athletes who are consuming a diet similar to that of the general population may have average intakes as low as 4g carbohydrate per kg body weight per day. Yet it has been shown by some researchers that intakes of 8g per kg body weight per day are still insufficient to prevent a significant reduction in muscle glycogen concentration after five days of hard training. This not only justifies the need to consume adequate amounts of carbohydrate but also the need for more frequent rest days

---

Estimated Daily Carbohydrate Requirements

Up to one hour of moderate intensity exercise or unlimited low intensity exercise per day: 5 to 7g carbohydrate per kg body weight.

Two or more hours of hard training a day: 7 to 10g carbohydrate per kg body weight.

---

between periods of high intensity training to allow the muscle glycogen levels to recover completely.

A 70 kg (11 st.) athlete doing several days of hard training needs to aim for a daily carbohydrate intake of 560 to 700g. Armed with information about the carbohydrate content of different foods, the task is then to build up the day's diet (meals, snacks and drinks) to reach the required carbohydrate intake in each 24-hour period. This is no mean task. When there are several days separating training or exercise sessions, a diet containing 5g carbohydrate per kg body weight a day should be sufficient to replace muscle glycogen stores.

Timing of Carbohydrate Intake

The time when the carbohydrate is eaten is also important. Glycogen is restored in the muscles at a rate of 5 per cent per hour after exercise. However, glycogen resynthesis during the first few hours after training has finished is inversely proportional to the amount of glycogen in the muscles and during the first two hours after exercise, glycogen is restored at the faster rate of 7 per cent.

Athletes should be encouraged to eat and/or drink carbohydrate-rich items as soon after exercise as is practical to make sure that glycogen replacement proceeds at a maximal rate. Here the goal to aim for is 1g carbohydrate per kg body weight within the first two hours and to start consuming this amount as early as possible – in the changing or dressing room rather than waiting to get home. It is important to avoid foods with a high fat content as fat can suppress appetite and consequently limit carbohydrate intake. This is particularly important if an athlete is intending to eat a meal rather than a snack immediately after a training session. (Note that the 1g carbohydrate per kg body weight required for immediate refuelling should be included within the total 24-hour requirement.)

Glycaemic Index and the Athlete

The glycaemic index (GI) of foods is simply a ranking of foods based on their immediate effect on blood sugar levels, not an indication of their nutritional value. Carbohydrate foods that are digested quickly have the highest GI factors whereas those that are digested more slowly will release glucose gradually into the blood stream. After exercise it is important to refuel as quickly as possible and it would seem sensible to encourage the use of high GI foods at this time and if appropriate, during exercise too. Similarly, low to moderate GI foods could be used before exercise to provide a more sustained source of carbohydrate.

Consuming carbohydrate during prolonged exercise can help to top-up the progressively depleting stores of muscle glycogen and therefore prolong the time before the onset of fatigue and the resulting dip in exercise capacity and performance. Whatever is consumed during exercise must be easily digested and absorbed and therefore available to provide a rapid source of energy. Also, no athlete wants to have the sensation of something swishing around in the stomach while exercising. Commercial sports drinks and energy bars, which tend to be popular choices amongst athletes for energy supply during exercise, are likely to produce

---

Glycaemic Index and Performance

Before exercise. Low GI carbohydrate-rich meals should be eaten, especially before endurance events.

During exercise. Moderate to high GI carbohydrate-rich drinks and food, if appropriate, should be consumed.

After exercise. High GI carbohydrate-rich drinks, snacks and meals should be consumed.

moderate to high glycaemic responses by the nature of their ingredients.

The GI may be a characteristic that could favour the choice of one food or drink above another for an athlete. However, there are other factors to be considered such as the nutritional balance of the food, as well as the cost, taste and practicality of the food (does it travel well, melt in warm weather, or need to be prepared in some way). Athletes must feel comfortable with the drinks and foods that they consume before, during and after exercise. Meals, snacks and drinks must be chosen to meet the needs of the athlete in various situations and certainly not chosen on the basis of the glycaemic index alone.

Sugar Before Exercise

Athletes are often advised not to consume sugar before exercise. This is based on one piece of research carried out in 1979 which showed that consuming 75g of glucose (300 kcal) thirty minutes before exercise reduced cycling time to exhaustion. The results were explained like this. The glucose caused the pancreas to put out large amounts of insulin which had the effect of lowering the blood sugar level and pushing the glucose into the muscles. The glucose level was further lowered when the muscles began to use blood glucose at the start of exercise. The overall lowering of blood sugar was thought to be responsible for the fatigue and subsequent drop in endurance performance.

However, subsequent research on pre-feeding with carbohydrate during the sixty-minute period before exercise has not backed up this finding. In five studies no adverse effect was observed and in five other studies performance was actually improved by the feeding.

Sugar During Exercise

When carbohydrate is consumed during exercise, it provides an extra source of fuel for the exercising muscles. It does not seem to change the rate of utilization of muscle glycogen, but provides some more fuel as blood glucose.

Hypoglycaemia

This is a condition when the blood glucose level drops below normal levels. Hypoglycaemia has become a popular diagnosis for a variety of otherwise undiagnosable symptoms including tiredness and depression. A very small percentage of the general public does experience genuine hypoglycaemia. Normally the movement of blood glucose into the muscles after ingestion of a meal or snack is very finely controlled by the production of the right amount of insulin to bring the blood glucose level back to normal. In this small group, however, the blood sugar level returns to normal very quickly after eating, so quickly that more insulin is produced than is needed. As a result, more sugar is removed from the blood stream causing the level to drop below normal, resulting in hypoglycaemia.

Many of the symptoms of hypoglycaemia are similar to those often related to stress such as sweating, palpitations, anxiety and weakness. Some include bad temper and poor concentration. A true diagnosis can only be made by a blood test carried out when the symptoms are actually present, in other words when the blood glucose level would be expected to be low.

Athletes who are medically diagnosed with hypoglycaemia should take preventative measures by eating regular meals and never missing breakfast, particularly if taking part in an early morning training session. They should try to eat at least every three hours and include low GI carbohydrate foods at all meals and snack occasions. They should mix high GI with low GI carbohydrate foods to give an overall moderate GI and avoid eating high GI carbohydrate-rich foods on their own as a snack.

Good Sources of Carbohydrate

√ = First choice foods (suitable for mealtimes)
R = Ideal for refuelling and snacks

√   Breakfast cereals – any variety (not necessarily whole grain) including hot cereals such as porridge. Many varieties can be eaten dry as a quick snack.

R√   Bread (white, wholemeal, granary, white soft grain, pitta bread, French bread, baguettes, rolls, baps, bagels, ciabatta and other continental types), muffins (English not American), crumpets, pikelets, naan, chappatis, potato cakes, raisin bread, malt loaf, fruit loaf, rye bread, tea breads, pancakes.

√   Crispbreads, water biscuits, oatcakes, rice cakes and matzos.

√   Pasta and noodles (all shapes and colours, fresh and dried).

√   Rice (all types).

√   Polenta, couscous, bulgar wheat, millet and other grain products.

√   Potatoes (mostly as boiled, mashed or jacket (old or new)), sweet potatoes, yam, cassava, plantains.

R   Popcorn (sugared not buttered).

√   Pizza bases (preferably deep pan or thin Italian style). However the topping may push up the fat content. Lower fat choices include ham and pineapple, vegetarian or ham and tomato.

√   Beans (baked, butter, red kidney, chickpeas, barlotti, cannelloni, mixed), peas, lentils, sweetcorn, pearl barley.

√   Root vegetables (carrots, parsnips, swedes, turnip, sweet potatoes, beetroot).

R√   Fruit (all sorts: fresh, dried, canned, cooked).

R   Cereal bars (some may have quite high fat contents).

R√   Jam, marmalade, honey, fruit spreads, golden syrup, maple syrup, molasses, black treacle.

R   Twiglets, sesame sticks, Japanese rice crackers, breadsticks, pretzels.

R   Biscuits ('plainer' varieties contain less fat, for example Jaffa cakes, fig rolls, Garibaldi, rich tea, plain digestives, McVitie's Go Ahead range of products, Jacob's Vitelinea range).

R   Cakes, such as currant buns, iced fruit buns, Chelsea buns, plain or fruit scones, fruit cake, gingerbread, parkin, jam-filled Swiss roll, flapjacks, McVitie's Cake Bars and other similar 'simple or plain' cakes.

R   Kellogg's Pop Tarts, Nutrigrain bars, Rice Krispie Squares and cereal and milk or yoghurt bars.

√   Puddings such as fruit crumbles, bread pudding, milk puddings (for example rice puddings, Mullerice), jelly and custard, banana and custard, meringue.

√   Yoghurt (plain and fruit). Mullerlight is sold in larger pots!

√   Milk and milk shakes.

R√   Sweetened soft drinks (squash, cordial, canned).

R√   Fruit juice and vegetable juice.

R   Chocolate bars (note the fat content of some varieties: ideally there should be at least three times as much carbohydrate as fat).

R   Sugar confectionery such as jelly beans, jelly babies, jelly tots, boiled sweets, liquorice allsorts, wine gums.

√   Sugar, added to drinks and breakfast cereals.

R   Commercial sports drinks such as Lucozade Sport, Isostar, Gatorade, Boots Isotonic, High5 Isotonic, Maxim Electrolyte.

R   Carbohydrate supplements (glucose polymers) such as Maxim, High Five Energy Source, PSP22.

Building Up the Carbohydrate Intake

An athlete may find the advice to eat a high carbohydrate diet daunting. After all, such a diet is not a typical Western diet. There are a wide variety of suitable carbohydrate foods that could be included but there is always a tendency to build the diet around a limited number of foods, such as breakfast cereal and sandwiches. Choosing foods that are enjoyed will help. Athletes should open their eyes to the huge variety of foods that are available and try something new.

Foods may be chosen because of nutritional misconceptions rather than for their appeal. For example, the general public is being encouraged to include more dietary fibre in the daily diet for health reasons, for example by eating plenty of whole grain cereals, wholemeal bread and brown rice. By their very nature, these foods are filling and will probably limit consumption so that the requirements of an athlete with high carbohydrate demands may not be met. Eating foods that are enjoyed will lead to a better intake so that requirements can be met.

Snacking is often seen as something to be avoided. This, again, may be appropriate advice for the sedentary individual but for those with high energy and carbohydrate requirements, eating little and often rather than having large infrequent meals is often the only way to meet requirements. It is not a crime to eat between meals and adopt a 'grazing' eating pattern.

Practical Ways to Increase the Carbohydrate Intake

Increasing the carbohydrate content of the diet is not just about knowing which foods to eat: there are also many practical ways of increasing the intake with foods that are already usually included in the diet. For example having two thin slices of bread from a large loaf will on average provide 29g of carbohydrate. Just changing to a thick sliced loaf can increase the carbohydrate intake to 41g.

Every meal and snack should be based around a carbohydrate-rich food. It should be the biggest portion of every meal with other foods added to it. This means adding the filling to the sandwich, sauce to the pasta, curry to the rice, tuna and sweetcorn to the jacket potato. The continental habit of eating bread as well as pasta, rice or potatoes with the main meal could be adopted. A loaf or rolls can be freshened up by wrapping in foil and putting in a preheated oven for five minutes or by using the microwave.

Jam, marmalade, honey and fruit spreads provide carbohydrate, as sugars, but no fat. They should be spread thickly and fat (such as margarine or butter) thinly, or not at all.

Potatoes boiled, mashed or baked in their skins are low in fat, chips are not. Thick-cut oven varieties with a low fat content (usually around 5 per cent sunflower oil) are the best chip choice. Add potatoes to soups and salads. Sweet potatoes, plantains and cassava have high carbohydrate contents and can make a change from potatoes.

Rice is a good source of carbohydrate although many people find it difficult to cook. The more expensive parboiled varieties are easier to cook. Brown rice takes a little longer to cook than white rice and requires more water, but it does not clump together as easily as white rice.

Pasta dishes can be given more variety by trying out different shapes and colours. Throwing in some herbs or spices to the cooking pasta or rice can also help to add extra interest. Extra pasta or rice cooked for the evening meal can be made into a salad for lunch the next day.

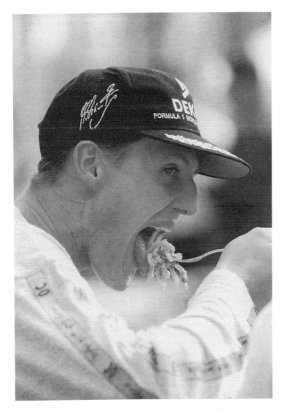

Michael Schumacher eating at the 1995 Pacific Grand Prix.

Experiment with different grains such as bulgar wheat, couscous and polenta – all available in quickly prepared forms.

Breakfast cereals are a good source of carbohydrate and can be eaten at any time for a snack (such as a late night supper) not just at breakfast time. Breakfast cereal and fruit juice complement each other. Both provide carbohydrate and the vitamin C in the juice helps the absorption of iron from the cereal. Fresh or dried fruit (especially bananas) added to a bowl of breakfast cereal pushes up the carbohydrate content.

There are lots of varieties of canned beans, peas and lentils which can be used to boost the carbohydrate content of soups, sauces and salads. Baked beans, red kidney beans, borlotti beans, cannellini beans, chickpeas and sweetcorn can be added to canned vegetable or minestrone soups, to tomato sauces with pasta or to curry sauces with rice. Baked beans on toast makes a quick and easy snack or light meal with a high carbohydrate content, and warm pitta bread could be used for a change. Frozen pitta bread can be warmed from frozen quickly in a toaster or under the grill.

A low fat milkshake made with skimmed or semi-skimmed milk, low fat yoghurt (plain or fruit) and a banana is quick to prepare and high in carbohydrate.

Meeting Carbohydrate Requirements

For some athletes, particularly those not involved in a regular training and competition programme, the advice given so far will be enough to ensure that glycogen stores are maintained and that fatigue and injuries do not lessen their enjoyment of their sport or exercise sessions. Others who train more regularly will want to ensure that they are meeting their carbohydrate requirement for the amount of exercise they are doing.

As far as the carbohydrate content of the diet is concerned, athletes need to aim for a total intake and within that total make sure that the refuelling requirement is also met. Equipped with information about portions of food and drink that provide 50g of carbohydrate and the carbohydrate content of items that would be suitable for immediate refuelling, the total carbohydrate intake can be built up.

Filling Up on the Way Home

For refuelling to be carried out efficiently, a certain amount of planning will be necessary on the part of the athlete. Suitable food and drink may be provided at the training venue,

Portions of Food Providing Approximately 50g of Carbohydrate

Breakfast Cereals

Food	Weight (Approx)	Household Measure
Porridge oats	75g	5 tablespoons
Wholewheat biscuits	65g	3 or 4 biscuits
Muesli	70g	5 tablespoons
Cornflake-type cereals	60g	10 tablespoons

Breads and Bakery Goods

Food	Weight (Approx)	Household Measure
Bread, large, medium sliced	100g	3 slices
Bread, large, thick sliced	100g	2½ slices
Bagel	70g	1
Rolls	100g	2
Baps (very large rolls)	100g	1
Pitta bread, large	95g	1
Crumpets	125g	3
Fruit scone	100g	2
Currant buns	100g	2
Malt loaf	100g	2½ slices
Raisin and lemon pancakes		3 pancakes

Cereals and Grains

Food	Weight (Approx)	Household Measure
Pasta (cooked)	225g (70g uncooked)	8 tablespoons
Rice (cooked)	175g (60g uncooked)	4 heaped tablespoons
Canned spaghetti in tomato sauce	400g	large can
Noodles	75g	1 sheet
Pizza base (thick)		½ large (9in)

Potatoes

Food	Weight (Approx)	Household Measure
Boiled	300g	5 egg sized
Jacket	175g	1 medium (with skin)
Mashed	325g	7 heaped tablespoons
Oven chips	175g	approx 20

Beans, Peas and Lentils

Food	Weight (Approx)	Household Measure
Baked beans	325g	8 tablespoons
Red kidney beans	280g	8 tablespoons
Chickpeas	310g	9 tablespoons
Sweetcorn (canned)	300g	10 tablespoons

Puddings

Food	Weight (Approx)	Household Measure
Rice pudding, low fat (canned)	425g	Whole can
Custard, low fat ready to serve	425g	Whole can
Ice-cream	225g	4 scoops
Arctic roll	150g	3 slices
Mullerice	250g	1¼ pots
Waitrose peach and banana smooth and fruity drink	330ml	one drink

Fruit

Food	Weight (Approx)	Household Measure
Apples		4 medium
Bananas		2 large
Dried apricots	100g	15
Dried dates	100g	7
Figs	100g	5
Raisins	70g	2½ tablespoons
Sultanas	70g	2½ tablespoons

Cereal and Breakfast Bars

Food	Household Measure
Jordan's Fruesli bars	2½
Jordan's Original bars	2½
Kellogg's Nutrigrains	2
Kellogg's Squares	2
McVitie's Go Ahead caramel crisp	3
McVitie's Go Ahead apple bakes	2
Jacob's Vitalinea chocolate orange fruit bar	2

Cakes and Biscuits

Food	Household Measure
Sainsbury's lemon slice	3
Chocolate mini Swiss roll	3
McVitie's cake bars	2 to 3
Mr Kipling mini Battenbergs	2
Plain digestives	5
Fig rolls	4 to 5
Ginger nut biscuits	7
Jaffa cakes	6
Iced gems	2 bags (30g)

Savoury Snacks

Food	Weight (Approx)	Household Measure
Twiglets	75g	1½ bag (50g)
Pretzels	60g	⅓ bag (175g)

Confectionery

Food	Weight (Approx)
Mars	1 standard bar
Milky Way	3 bars (26g)
Crunchie	2 standard bars
Jelly Beans	½ 125g pack
Jelly Babies	¼ 225g pack
Turkish Delight	1¼ bars

sandwiches squashed at the bottom of the kit bag are not going to be very tempting. Nor will crumbled biscuits, melted chocolate confectionery (suitable items of course) or a leaky pot of yoghurt encourage an athlete who has little appetite after a hard session. Many athletes will probably stop off at a garage on their way home and this can offer ideal re-fuellers but also quite a lot of inappropriate items as well.

Crisps and Similar Snacks

Crisps do contain reasonable amounts of vitamin C and some fibre but they also have a high fat content. Low fat versions have around a third less fat than regular crisps. Highly flavoured items may repeat later which could be a problem in some circumstances. Best choices in this group are Twiglets, pretzels or Japanese rice crackers.

Chocolate

Chocolate does contain magnesium, iron and vitamin B_2 and milk chocolate contains calcium too. There is plenty of carbohydrate in the form of simple sugars but a lot of the energy or calories comes from fat. Ordinary milk chocolate provides 45 per cent of energy as carbohydrate and 52 per cent as fat. Chocolate bars that contain nuts, caramel or toffee tend to have even higher fat contents. The nutritional information will show which bars give most carbohydrate for least fat. Best choices are Crunchie bars and Turkish Delight (the type with chocolate of course).

Sweets

A large percentage of sweets are more or less pure carbohydrate. Toffees and chocolate-coated sweets will of course have higher fat contents. Those that have a jelly nature to them will have a small amount of protein (from the gelatin) but this is not a significant advantage as gelatin is not a high nutritive

but an athlete training at a new venue should never assume that there will be suitable food and drink. Taking refuellers in the kit bag is the safest option, although it is important that the chosen items travel well. Bananas or value protein. Sucking boiled sweets or peppermints will keep energy levels topped up a little and keep the mouth refreshed but constant sweet popping can play havoc with the teeth. Best choices are any that appeal.

Biscuits

Plain dry savoury biscuits such as water biscuits, crackers or crispbreads are probably not going to be an athlete's choice from an enjoyment or convenience factor, though they are high in carbohydrate and low in fat. Cheesy biscuits like Cheddars and most chocolate biscuits will be too high in fat for effective refuelling. Non-chocolate biscuits will provide more carbohydrate for less fat with the exception of creams and shortbread varieties. Anything with 'butter' in the name will also have a higher fat content. Best choices are biscuits like ginger nuts, rich tea biscuits, fig rolls and of course Jaffa cakes.

Cereal Bars

Cereal bars can be a good choice, but it is important to read the labels. There is no easy way of knowing which are higher in carbohydrate and which contain perhaps too much fat unless you check the information provided. Best choices are Fruesli bars and Nutrigrains.

Sandwiches and Rolls

Sandwiches and rolls are becoming standard items in garages although information on the packaging may not include nutritional content. The bread will provide plenty of carbohydrate, the spread some fat but the biggest variable will be the filling. Best choices for fillings include salad, tuna or salmon, cheese, chicken, lean ham or prawns, but most will contain high fat mayonnaise.

What Else?

Plain popcorn is a possibility and certainly fruit, especially bananas if they are available.

Buns and cakes might be fine, particularly scones, currant buns, malt bread and banana bread. Some flapjacks and crispie cakes are not too high in fat but pastry (fruit pies, Eccles cakes and sausage rolls) is certainly not the ideal choice. A sports drink will also help in refuelling.

Carbohydrate Supplements

Athletes involved in regular intense training may find it difficult to consume sufficient carbohydrate to meet their requirements. The training load may affect appetite, and the athlete may find the stress of trying to eat enough pasta, bread, etc., to be such a chore that he or she loses interest in food and ends up eating even less. Lack of time between training sessions may limit food choices and gastric discomfort may result if a bulky meal is eaten close to training.

The use of concentrated sources of carbohydrate in the form of powders, drinks and energy bars may be the answer for some athletes, helping to top-up the intake from meals and snacks. These products must be viewed as supplements to, and not replacements for, a suitable diet. They will not turn a junk diet into a healthy well-balanced diet and they will not be needed if the athlete is already eating sufficient carbohydrate-rich foods. Adding high-energy products to a diet that already contains enough energy will result in weight increase rather than an improvement in performance. High-energy products can be used before and after training sessions but are not usually appropriate for consuming during a session as they can affect fluid replacement.

Energy or sports bars may be of use for some athletes. They are convenient, travel well and appear to be digested easily. The same of course could equally be said of many, much cheaper, cereal bars. Some bars have a higher fat content, following the sparing glycogen theory (*see* page 67), and athletes should check the composition of the bar to make sure that it is suitable.

FAT

Athletes have an increased demand for energy (calories). On a weight-for-weight basis, fat provides more than twice the number of calories than carbohydrate or protein. However adding large amounts of fat into the diet is not the best way to meet the energy requirement. Fat, stored as adipose tissue, does provide fuel, particularly in light intensity exercise and in prolonged endurance exercise but even in the leanest of athletes there is never any shortage and no risk of running out. It is the fuel stores of carbohydrate or glycogen that are the limiting factor.

Fat Requirements

Fat is needed in the diet. It has many important functions and athletes should never attempt to follow a 'no-fat' diet. However in order to achieve the required intake of carbohydrate and protein while maintaining body weight it will be necessary to ensure a low intake of fat. Most athletes will be able to do this by learning which foods contain relatively large amounts of fat and by following simple practical guidelines. Some athletes, not content with counting grams of carbohydrate and protein, like to count fat grams.

The following table is intended to give an idea of possible fat intakes for given total energy intakes but it must be stressed that athletes should not become paranoid about counting. Also, the assumption should not be made that an intake of 20 per cent of total calories from fat is always better than 30 per cent. For example athletes who are battling to prevent weight loss will need more fat than

How Much Fat is Needed?			
Energy needs per day (kcal)	*Amount of fat in the diet (g)*		
	20% fat	25% fat	30% fat
1,500	30	40	50
2,000	45	55	65
2,500	55	70	85
3,000	65	85	100
3,500	80	100	115
4,000	90	110	135
(Figures rounded to the nearest 5.)			

athletes who need to lose body fat. It should also be remembered that some foods that are high in fat can also be very good sources of essential nutrients, for example cheese. It is therefore important not to exclude such items from the diet but rather to look for low fat varieties or use smaller portions.

Reducing Fat in the Diet

Athletes need to know which foods contribute fat in the diet and to aim to limit the occasions that they consume such high fat foods (*see* Chapter 1). There are also many practical ways that fat intakes can be reduced without making major changes to the overall diet.

Choose a low fat spread rather than butter, hard margarine or soft margarine but spread it thinly (particularly if the amount of bread being eaten increases). Sometimes it is not necessary to put fat on bread or toast, for example when preparing baked beans on toast, when making peanut butter, chocolate spread or honey sandwiches and when eating the tasty continental breads.

Switch from whole milk to semi-skimmed or skimmed milk. Both have slightly more calcium and protein than whole milk but much less fat. Use skimmed milk in cooking and semi-skimmed in drinks and on cereals. (Dried milk food labels should be read carefully to make sure that the milk powder does not contain extra fat as added vegetable fat).

Avoid anything but occasional use of cream, evaporated milk and condensed milk. Single cream contains significantly less fat than double cream. Low fat yoghurt, *fromage frais* (labelled less than 1 per cent fat) and 0 per cent fat Quark and 0 per cent fat Greek yoghurt are good substitutes for cream or mayonnaise and can be used to make 'creamy' sauces for pasta, to top off jacket potatoes or as a basis for salad dressings. Artificial creams made from vegetable oils have just as much fat as dairy cream (unless of course specified as fat-reduced or low fat).

Use half fat hard cheeses instead of full fat varieties, or use less of a strongly flavoured full fat cheese. Curd cheese or low fat soft cheese can always be used instead of cream cheese in sandwiches and cooking. Low fat soft cheese can be melted down gently to make a creamy but low fat sauce for pasta or vegetables. The staple of the serious dieter, cottage cheese, now comes in many flavours to add a little more variety to an otherwise bland product. Grated cheese goes further than slices in a sandwich.

Make salad dressings with low fat natural yoghurt, herbs, spices, tomato juice, vinegar or lemon juice rather than salad cream or mayonnaise.

Avoid over-cooking vegetables so that they retain flavour and thus avoid the need to top them with butter or margarine before serving.

Cut down (but not necessarily cut out completely) crisps, chocolate, pastries and 'rich' cakes and biscuits. Fruit (fresh and dried), sandwiches with low fat fillings, 'plain' cakes and biscuits (current buns, scones, tea bread, crumpets, rich tea biscuits, fig rolls, plain digestives) are all suitable low fat snack foods.

Eat fish more often and grill, microwave,

steam or bake it rather than deep-frying in batter. Fish cakes and fish fingers can also be grilled rather than fried. Choose fish canned in brine, water or tomatoes rather than in oil. Alternatively, drain off as much of the oil as possible.

Chicken and turkey are low in fat as long as the skin is discarded. Most of the fat is found underneath the skin and comes off when the skin is removed. If preferred, the skin can be removed after cooking. Buy the leanest cuts of meat and trim off any visible fat. Farming and butchering techniques nowadays have resulted in a considerable fat reduction, and lean meat should certainly no longer be considered a high fat food. Use smaller amounts of meat and replace it with vegetables, potatoes and beans, peas and lentils. This will not only keep the fat content very low but also boost the carbohydrate content of the meal.

Microwave, steam, poach, boil, grill or stir-fry food rather than frying it in order to make large savings in fat content. Using non-stick pans can eliminate the need to add any fat or at least no more than a spray of oil. When roasting food, using a trivet or stand allows the fat to drip out. Use as little oil as possible in cooking by measuring the oil rather than just pouring it from the container. Stir-frying in a wok requires much less fat than shallow or deep-frying.

Any fat that appears from mince or casserole meat during cooking should be skimmed off or mopped up with a piece of kitchen paper. Up to 40 per cent of the fat content can be removed this way. The fat content of mince can be reduced by heating the mince, adding cold water, allowing to cool slightly and pouring off the fat with the water, then cooking the mince in the usual way. When making gravy from meat juices (so getting the benefit of the vitamins that leach out in cooking), drain off as much fat as possible or add a few ice cubes to the pan – as the fat becomes solid it can easily be removed. Alternatively, use a gravy pourer which is designed to leave the fat behind.

Meat products such as sausages and beef-burgers can be fatty so should not be eaten too often. Grilling low fat varieties will keep the fat content down. Meat pies, sausage rolls and pasties contain large amounts of fat in both the meat and pastry. Intakes of these items should be limited to the occasional rather than the regular.

The fat content of pastry items can be reduced by choosing items with only one layer (top or bottom pastry crust), lattice top pies, fruit crumbles instead of fruit pies and filo pastry instead of other types of pastry.

Chips should not have a regular place in an athlete's diet but there is nothing wrong with the occasional portion at an appropriate time (not as a pre-competition meal for instance). Lowest fat contents are achieved by choosing thick, non-crinkle oven chips (usually with no more than 5 per cent sunflower oil). Thin-cut and crinkle-cut chips absorb more fat as their surface area is larger. 'Roast' potatoes can be made by parboiling, brushing lightly with oil and crisping in a pre-heated oven.

Check food labels and choose lower fat products instead of traditional high fat ones. These are often flagged up as low or lower fat but it is always sensible to check to see what the saving actually is and what the energy content is too. Athletes needing to lose weight may otherwise chose a product that on a calorie basis is not significantly different from other products not labelled as low fat.

Is There a Role for High Fat Diets?

There is no good evidence to suggest that performance can be improved by increasing fat intake or similarly decreasing carbohydrate intake, with perhaps the exception of the ultra-endurance athlete. In comparison, there is no shortage of evidence that adequate carbohydrate intakes are necessary for maximizing performance. Fat can be utilized in low intensity exercise but fat oxidation cannot supply energy fast enough when exercise intensity is greater than about 60 per cent VO2max (moderate intensity exercise). Eating too much fat also tends to decrease carbohydrate intake so that muscle glycogen stores are not maintained satisfactorily. From a health point of view, high fat diets are associated with heart disease, stroke, some forms of cancer and of course overweight and obesity.

Fat loading is claimed to help athletes to burn fat and so spare the limited supply of glycogen which in turn can enhance the capacity for endurance exercise. This sounds all very well in theory but in practice, achieving a significant increase in available fat through increased fat consumption does not appear to happen.

Indeed, from the available literature, based on human studies, it seems that ingestion of a high fat diet for three to five days leads to a deterioration in endurance performance compared with endurance performance on a high carbohydrate diet. From one to four weeks, a high fat diet in combination with training does not reduce endurance performance compared with a high carbohydrate diet but neither does it improve it. However, after seven weeks on the regime, endurance performance was markedly better on the high carbohydrate diet compared with the high fat diet. In addition, high fat diets take longer to digest, hence the avoidance of high fat foods in a pre-exercise meal. There also does not seem to be any benefit gained when an athlete switches to a high carbohydrate diet after a long-term adaptation to a high fat diet, compared to maintaining a constant high carbohydrate intake.

Aerobic training of course does increase an athlete's ability to use fat, primarily the intra-muscular triglyceride stored directly within the muscle fibres, as a fuel.

Do Medium Chain Triglycerides Have a Role?

One possible way to increase fatty acid oxidation during prolonged exercise, thus sparing the limited supply of muscle glycogen, might be to consume fat to provide additional fuel. Fats consumed in the normal diet tend to have large chemical structures which take a long time to digest and absorb. Apart from the potential discomfort of consuming fat during exercise, any benefits are unlikely to be realised, unless exercising for a very prolonged period of time, as absorption will not have taken place by the time the athlete stops exercising.

Medium chain triglycerides (MCT) are semi-synthetic oil mixtures, prepared from natural coconut oil. MCT have physical characteristics different to those of the longer chain triglycerides found in food and these have made them interesting in clinical nutrition situations and now also in the sports nutrition setting. They are water soluble and emptied from the stomach, digested, absorbed and oxidized rapidly. Unfortunately, 30g of MCT, equivalent to 250kcal, is all that most people can tolerate. Such an intake does not affect muscle glycogen breakdown and itself only contributes 7 per cent of the total energy expenditure of exercise. Ingesting larger amounts may result in stomach cramps and diarrhoea ranging in intensity from mild to crippling. Such an intake is unlikely to figure as a significant source of fuel for athletes. If larger amounts could be tolerated, MCT might well prove to be a beneficial supplement for endurance performance.

The Zone Diet

The Zone is a popular dietary regimen promoted by Barry Sears in his book (*The Zone*). He claims that 'the Zone' is a physiological condition achieved by consuming food in the precise proportions of 40 per cent of total energy as carbohydrate, 30 per cent as protein and 30 per cent as fat at each of three daily meals and two daily snacks. The theory behind the 40:30:30 diet is that people should lower their level of insulin by eating a high protein, moderate fat and low carbohydrate diet. High carbohydrate intakes, it is claimed cause the body to produce too much insulin which can cause weight gain. There is in fact no scientific evidence to suggest that carbohydrates stimulate appetite and lead to more fat storage and weight gain. Regardless of their source, excess calories cause weight gain. Contrary to the Zone 'carbo-hell' theory, the health benefits of carbohydrates are well-documented by scientific studies. From the athlete's point of view, following such a diet will make it very difficult to train or compete. Low stores of muscle glycogen will cause fatigue and necessitate a reduction in exercise intensity level.

The diet centres primarily around an intake of 1.8 to 2.2g protein per kg fat free mass (total body weight minus body fat weight), which is higher than recommendations for both endurance and strength/speed athletes. The aim of the protein content of the Zone diet is to maintain energy levels and aid recovery. Certainly a novel idea but how valid? Protein can be used to supply energy, particularly when there is a shortage of carbohydrate. However using protein for energy is inefficient (and expensive) and high protein diets as already explained are not recommended because of a number of health implications.

Once the protein requirement has been

The Zone Diet Guidelines

All meals and snacks must maintain the ratio of one to one carbohydrate and protein.

Food will need to be weighed in order to achieve the prescribed ratios.

Eat more fruit and vegetables than bread, pasta or rice.

Protein choices must be low in fat.

Fat intake must be primarily monounsaturates (olive oil).

Drink at least half a pint of water (flavoured if necessary with sugar-free squash) with every meal and snack.

Eat regularly and never go more than five hours without food.

Craving sugar and feeling hungry after a meal means that too much carbohydrate has been eaten.

---

calculated, the energy value of the protein can be calculated. This must represent 30 per cent of the total energy intake. Using the Zone Diet energy intakes for carbohydrate (40 per cent) and fat (30 per cent), the total energy value of the diet can now be calculated. This reveals the Zone Diet to be in most cases a low energy diet. The claim that athletes can improve performance by having a diet of 40 per cent of total energy from carbohydrates within a total energy intake of less than 2,000kcal has not been substantiated by reliable scientific evidence.

PROTEIN

Protein and its effect on performance and body composition has been a topic of great interest to athletes for a long time. This belief in protein goes back to ancient times when athletes ate raw meat in the hope of increasing their own muscle mass. Many athletes today, especially those participating in power sports

and strength training, still believe that a high protein diet increases muscle mass and supplies extra energy, thus enhancing athletic performance. These beliefs are further encouraged by the claims made by some manufacturers of protein and amino acid supplements.

Protein as a Source of Energy

If the diet is low in carbohydrate, there is a greater use of protein as an energy source. This of course leaves little protein for its major function of muscle repair and growth. In situations where energy demands are high and prolonged, as in endurance events, protein may provide a significant quantity of amino acids for use as an extra fuel source, on top of the supply of carbohydrate and fat. If this is so, an inadequate intake of protein (and/or too frequent training) could lead to losses of protein from liver and muscles which would eventually impair athletic performance.

To examine the use of amino acids as a fuel during exercise, the amino acid leucine has been used as a tracer and increased oxidation of leucine during aerobic exercise has been observed. The size of the increase is dependent on the intensity and duration of the exercise and also on the athlete's level of training. The largest increase occurs during exhaustive endurance exercise with untrained individuals. With training, leucine oxidation decreases, thus the need for leucine and therefore protein is greater for those who are starting endurance training. There is a need for more protein to meet the requirement of the increase in muscle mass, red blood cells, myoglobin and enzymes required for metabolism that is taking place at this time. In strength training, protein is not used as a fuel source.

Protein and Muscle Mass

Muscle mass is determined by the training effect and not by excessive intakes of dietary protein. Protein is important (after all it provides most of the structural elements of the muscle cell) but it is training that stimulates protein synthesis. Strength is proportional to the cross-sectional area of the muscle and this is related to increases in the diameter of the individual muscle fibres making up the muscle. As a result of training, there is an increase in amino acid transport into the muscle cells which enhances their incorporation in the muscle proteins. Not only does the muscle get stronger but also the tendons get thicker and the bone gets stronger, particularly where the tendon joins the bone. All these adaptations are obviously vital if the athlete is to avoid injury.

Anabolic steroids often cause a mismatch as muscle increase is not matched by tendon increase and this can result in injuries where the tendon joins the bone. To gain muscle mass, athletes must increase the workload on their muscles by a well-planned training programme and eat a diet that contains not only protein but also adequate energy.

Protein and Recovery From Exercise

There is a decrease in protein synthesis during strength training exercise but after exercise protein synthesis increases to a greater level than pre-exercise. This effect lasts for about twelve hours. Intakes of carbohydrate after exercise stimulate muscle growth by the action of insulin on protein synthesis. Addition of protein together with carbohydrate in the post-exercise recovery phase also increases protein synthesis. Protein increases the concentration of insulin in the blood to a greater extent than carbohydrate alone. A ratio of 3:1 for carbohydrate-protein supplementation after exercise has been suggested but the optimal mix has yet to be determined.

Protein Requirements

Current general recommendations for protein intake, set at 0.75g protein per kg body weight per day are based on a sedentary lifestyle and do not take into account the effects of regular exercise, which will require an increase in protein intake. Current evidence suggests that strength or speed athletes should consume about 1.7 to 1.8g protein per kg body weight per day and endurance athletes about 1.2 to 1.4g protein per kg body weight per day. Putting it into context, this is 100 to 212 per cent of the requirement of the average sedentary individual.

Food Portions Providing Approximately 20g of Protein		
Food	Weight (Approx)	Portion of Food
Beef, lamb, pork	75g	2 medium slices
Chicken	75g	1 small breast
Fish	100g	1 medium fillet
Fish fingers	135g	5 fingers
Tuna in brine	100g	1 small can
Prawns, boiled (no shell)	100g	approx 30 small prawns
Semi-skimmed milk	600ml	1 pint
Cheddar cheese, reduced fat	60g	2 matchbox-sized pieces
Eggs		3 size 2 eggs
Baked beans	400g	1 large can
Lentils, cooked or canned	265g	6½ tablespoons
Nuts	100g	100g bag
Seeds	100g	100g bag (6 tablespoons)
Tofu, steamed	250g	1 serving

However, this does not mean that athletes should be reaching for the nearest protein or amino acid supplement. Instead, they should be ensuring that they include a wide variety of protein-rich foods in their daily diet (*see* Chapter 1).

Eastern European countries tend to favour much higher intakes of protein. For general training, intakes of 2.2 to 2.6g protein per kg body weight per day are recommended with up to 4.0g protein per kg body weight per day for intense strength training. The aim is to maintain positive nitrogen balance and maximise strength gains. There is, however, inadequate evidence to endorse these recommendations.

Recommended intakes of protein for both strength/speed and endurance athletes can be met by a diet which consists of 12 to 15 per cent of energy from protein, unless the total energy intake is not enough. Assuming a 70kg (11 st) male athlete is maintaining his body weight (and therefore meeting his energy needs) on a daily intake of 3,500kcal. If 12 to 15 per cent of that energy is protein, he will be obtaining 105 to 132g protein from his diet which is equivalent to 1.5 to 1.9g protein/kg body weight/day. These levels of protein intake are not high when taken in relation to the increased energy intake needed for training.

Too Little Protein in the Diet

A few athletes are at risk of not getting enough protein. These include those who are restricting their food intake to lose excess body fat or to make weight for competition. Those who are fussy eaters may also be at risk of not eating enough protein. Endurance athletes sometimes include so much carbohydrate in their diet that the protein content of the diet becomes too low. Children who are particularly physically active can also be at risk

of not obtaining enough protein from their diet (*see* Chapter 8).

Poor protein intakes can lead to loss of muscle, slow recovery after exercise and, if protein intakes are chronically low, serious health implications.

Protein in the Diet

The safest and simplest way to maintain an adequate protein intake is to eat a wide variety of foods. Many sources of vegetable protein (peas, beans, lentils and nuts) contain large amounts of carbohydrate, dietary fibre, vitamins and minerals as well as protein and these foods should be included perhaps more often than in the average diet. Foods included in the diet primarily for their carbohydrate content also make significant contributions to the overall protein intake, not because they are particularly rich in protein but because they are eaten in large amounts. For example, four slices of bread, eight tablespoons of cooked pasta or twelve tablespoons of cooked rice will each provide 10g protein.

Muscle growth is stimulated only in the presence of adequate amino acids, so the intake of dietary protein should be spread throughout the day in order to maintain optimal blood amino acid levels.

Are Protein Supplements Necessary?

As energy intake increases to meet the extra energy costs of exercise, there is an automatic increase in protein intake. Protein supplements are therefore unlikely to be necessary. One pint of milk will provide a similar amount of protein to a serving of a protein supplement (which will often be based on milk protein) at a much lower price. A liquid meal replacement containing not only protein but also carbohydrate, minerals and vitamins may be useful if an athlete is having problems meeting energy requirements. Liquid meals are sometimes tolerated more easily than a greater quantity of solid food and could help the athlete who is trying to gain weight or at least prevent weight loss.

Can Excessive Protein Intakes be Harmful?

Protein intakes in excess of requirements need to be broken down for excretion from the body. This requires more water than the breakdown of carbohydrate or fat. With increasing protein breakdown, there is a need for an increased fluid intake to prevent dehydration. Excess protein intakes have been associated with possible kidney malfunction. However intakes of 2.0 to 2.2g protein per kg body weight per day do not appear to have any adverse effects on kidney function. There is no reliable data for intakes above these values, particularly for people with normal, healthy kidneys.

Protein-rich foods are generally the more expensive food items in the shopping trolley. Some can be major sources of fat as well as protein. Perhaps of greater concern is the use of amino acid supplements and the toxic effects on the body if excess individual amino acids are ingested.

VITAMINS

Many athletes regularly take vitamin supplements throughout training and competition, in the mistaken belief that extra vitamins will improve performance, perhaps by helping to the body to withstand the exertion of intensive, competitive training. It is true that many of the water-soluble vitamins are involved in the oxidation of carbohydrate and fat to provide energy but there is no evidence that taking large doses will release energy faster.

Folate and vitamin B_{12} are important in red blood cell formation but adding extra amounts of these to the diet will not stimulate the production of more red blood cells.

If there is a vitamin deficiency because requirements are not being met, then health and performance will suffer. Taking a supplement and ensuring that the diet from then on contains enough of the vitamin should result in an improvement in performance. However there is no evidence that taking extra vitamins on top of a perfectly adequate diet will have any positive effect on performance.

Many athletes experience tiredness, lethargy or heaviness in the legs and may assume this to be caused by lack of vitamins (many of the first signs of sub-clinical deficiencies of vitamins are very similar). More likely causes for these symptoms are inadequate energy, carbohydrate and/or fluid intakes. Alternatively, the cause may be over-training (for example by not including rest days in the schedule) so that there is incomplete recovery between training sessions. In all these cases, reaching for a vitamin supplement will not provide the answer.

Do Athletes Have a Greater Requirement for Vitamins?

There appears to be no value in consuming additional amounts of vitamins once the body's requirements are met. But what are an athlete's requirements? Surely with the increased energy requirement there must be a similar increase in vitamin requirement?

Theoretically, an increased requirement can be caused by decreased absorption by the digestive system, increased excretion in sweat, urine and faeces and increased turnover, as well as through a biochemical adaptation to training. However, there is little evidence to suggest that athletes excrete more vitamins in urine and faeces or that they have a higher turnover of vitamins than non-athletes do. Even vitamin loss through sweat is negligible. The 'assumed' increased requirements are most likely to be the result of biochemical adaptations to training. In most situations this increased requirement will be met by the diet alone, but not always.

Who is at Risk of Inadequate Intakes?

Some athletes lack the incentive to prepare meals and so rely heavily on convenience food and take-away meals with a minimum intake of fresh food, particularly fruit and vegetables. Others may not eat properly because of lack of time to shop, cook or even eat and so regularly skip meals. A diet predominantly made up of sugars and refined starches may have a low nutrient density and could lead to poor vitamin intake. Restricted vegetarian diets and severe weight reduction diets can also cause inadequate vitamin intake, as can general fussy eating. Some drugs (notably aspirin and other anti-inflammatory drugs taken regularly in large doses) and oral contraceptives interfere with the metabolism of certain vitamins. Excess alcohol and regular smoking also augment the requirements for some vitamins.

However, all of these are lifestyle issues, rather than an increase in the vitamin requirements for those undertaking regular exercise. A multi-vitamin supplement will never replace a healthy diet or make up for a poor one, but it can help to reduce the nutritional gaps in the diet.

Choosing and Using a Supplement

A multivitamin and/or mineral supplement is the best choice for all-round supplementation because it delivers nutrients in the right balance. A supplement providing no more than 100 per cent of the Recommended Daily Amount (RDA) for each vitamin or mineral should be chosen for topping-up or as an 'insurance policy' for the diet. A recognisable brand name will ensure the highest level of quality control.

Athletes should not combine different supplements without first seeking advice from their doctor, pharmacist, sports dietitian or the company manufacturing the supplement. Combining supplements can lead to over-dosing and an imbalance of nutrients. Supplements should only be taken in the amounts recommended on the pack by the manufacturer or retailer. It is not a case of more is better.

The time of day when they are taken is not important but they should be taken regularly. Many athletes find it best to get into a routine, for example by always taking the supplement with breakfast or the evening meal.

Supplements containing vitamin B_2 (riboflavin) can cause an athlete to produce bright yellow urine. (This vitamin is used in the food industry to colour food.) This can have implications when using urine colour as a sign of hydration status.

Supplements should normally be stored in a cool, dry place. There should be storage instructions on the packaging. The product and packaging should be tamper proof and sell-by dates should always be checked before purchase. The product should be comprehensively and accurately labelled for content, necessary safety warnings and precautions such as 'do not exceed stated dose', 'keep away from children' and so on. Access to professional advice should always be available when buying a health supplement. This may be at point of sale, supplied with the product or available on a telephone helpline.

RNI and RDA

Medical personnel, dietitians and nutritionists make use of the Reference Nutrient Intake figures (RNI) when assessing whether intakes of nutrients such as vitamins and minerals are adequate. Vitamin and mineral supplement labelling declarations on pack use the Recommended Daily Amount (RDA) figure from the Food Labelling Regulations of 1996 which may be higher or lower than the RNI figure for a particular nutrient. A supplement labelled as containing 100 per cent RDA levels of vitamin C (60mg) for example, would contain 150 per cent of the RNI figure for men and women (40mg).

Beware of Megadosing

Taking multiple doses of the RDA of some supplements, commonly known as 'megadosing', may have adverse effects which can result in harmful side effects. A high dose of vitamin A can lead to liver and bone damage and is linked to birth defects. High intakes of vitamin B_6 can lead to temporary nerve problems.

Taking high doses of some vitamins or minerals can interfere with the absorption of other nutrients which in time can lead to deficiencies. High intakes of iron can reduce absorption of zinc and too much zinc can interfere with copper absorption. Hence the advice is not to take cocktails of high doses of single vitamins or minerals.

Taking vitamin C in doses of 2 to 3g or more a day can cause diarrhoea and increase the risk of kidney stones in susceptible people. If very high doses of vitamin C are taken on a regular basis, it is possible to become dependent on the high intake. When the supplement is no longer taken, deficiency symptoms can then develop. In this case it is important to reduce the intake of the supplement gradually.

Upper Safe Levels for Long Term Use of Daily Vitamin Supplements	
Vitamin	*Upper Safe Level*
Vitamin A	2,300µg
Vitamin B_1	100mg
Vitamin B_2	200mg
Niacin	150mg
Vitamin B_6	100mg
Vitamin B_{12}	3000µg
Folic acid	400µg
Biotin	2,500µg
Pantothenic acid	1,000mg
Vitamin C	2,000mg
Vitamin D	10µg
Vitamin E	800mg

(Source: Council for Responsible Nutrition, an association of leading suppliers of food supplements and the European Federation of Associations of Health Product Manufacturers which represents specialist health product manufacturers in Europe.)

These intakes of vitamins are in addition to the amounts gained from the diet. The upper safe level for supplementation is an indication to consumers of consumption levels that it would be unwise to exceed. It is not a definition of levels that could be advocated to promote general health.

Many vitamins are soluble in water and excess intakes are lost in the urine. Some supplements simply do nothing more than produce expensive urine. Pregnant women should not take any vitamin and mineral supplements unless advised to do so by their doctor or ante-natal clinic, with the exception of folic acid. In this special case, women who may become pregnant or who are up to twelve weeks pregnant are recommended to take 400µg daily to reduce the risk of having a baby with a neural tube defect such as spina bifida.

A Warning Note

There are many other substances which have been classed as vitamins, packaged into neat tablets and swallowed in the belief that they will, among other things, improve health, protect against diseases, slow down the ageing process and aid athletic performance. However, some of them are not thought to be physiologically active and others, although accepted as active, are no longer termed vitamins. These 'rogue' vitamins include B$_4$ (adenine), B$_7$ (choline or vitamin J), B$_{13}$ (orotic acid) and B$_{15}$ (pangamic acid). Taking any of these substances as expensive supplements is unlikely to affect performance. Money would be better spent on buying a larger variety of foods, particularly fruit and vegetables.

Is There a Special Case for the Antioxidants?

Regular exercise may have positive effects on the immune system but there have also been some concerns raised that such benefits will be outweighed by the production of free radicals and oxidative stress which occur during exercise. These free radicals seem to be closely involved in tissue and cell damage induced by exercise. The level of free radical production may be overwhelming the body's ability to mop up the free radicals before they can do too much damage. This is more likely during prolonged aerobic exercise, resistance training or when antioxidant defence mechanisms are impaired.

Nutritional antioxidants include vitamins A (as the precursor beta-carotene), C and E. Supplementation with these vitamins does not appear to affect exercise performance directly but it may help in the recovery from exercise. The damage these free radicals do at the tissue and cellular level may be the cause of the muscle damage, soreness or inflammation that is often experienced after strenuous exercise. Thus there may be long-term benefits in taking an antioxidant supplement, particularly by those athletes who habitually have a low intake of fresh fruit and vegetables.

At the moment, it seems unlikely that supplementing with anything more than a simple multivitamin/mineral supplement or a supplement containing the antioxidant nutrients in doses similar to the RDA is needed. Evidence also suggests that those who exercise regularly are less prone to damage than those who participate in exercise in a more erratic and haphazard manner. An athlete following an intense, regular training programme may therefore benefit less from supplements than an individual exercising or participating in sport as and when time permits. Supplementation aside, all athletes would benefit from consuming at least five portions of fruit and vegetables on a daily basis as not only will this supply the antioxidant vitamins but also the phytochemicals which are also believed to have important antioxidant properties.

MINERALS

Minerals are essential nutrients and, like vitamins, must be supplied in the diet. However with the exception of calcium and iron, deficiencies are uncommon. The intake of calcium and iron, however, should be of concern to all athletes. This is especially so for female athletes because of the potential effect on health in later life as well as the immediate effect on performance (*see* Chapter 9). Unfortunately, the dietary practices adopted by many athletes are anything but helpful.

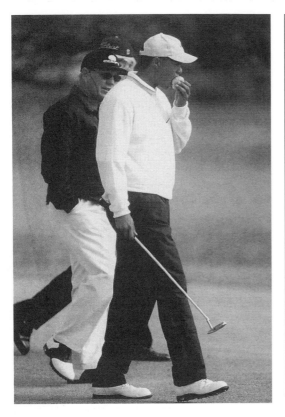

Tiger Woods takes a bite from an apple at the 1999 Open.

What are Portions of Fruit and Vegetables?

A portion could be:

- One large slice of a very large fruit (melon, pineapple).
- One medium fruit (apple, pear, orange).
- Two small fruit (plums, satsumas, kiwi fruit).
- One cup of grapes or of berries (raspberries, strawberries and so on).
- Two to three tablespoons of fruit salad (fresh, stewed or canned).
- One tablespoon of dried fruit.
- One glass of fruit juice.
- Two tablespoons of vegetables (fresh, frozen or canned).
- One dessert bowl of salad.

Potatoes count as carbohydrate foods, not vegetables, in this context. Fruit juice can only be counted once, regardless of the quantity and frequency of drinking.

Calcium

Almost ninety per cent of calcium is found in the bones. Bone is an active tissue, constantly changing as the result of the continual process of bone resorption and bone formation known as 'bone remodelling'. This process of remodelling continues throughout life but at different rates. Peak bone mass is the highest bone mass that is achieved in a person's lifetime and this is normally reached by the early thirties. After this time, resorption starts to exceed formation slightly with a resulting drop in bone mass with age. It appears that the rate of decline in bone mass with age is similar for all persons regardless of the peak bone mass achieved. Having a high peak bone mass will help to prevent or at least delay the onset of osteoporosis (brittle bone disease).

Physical activity exerts an anabolic effect on the skeleton. Bone density tends to be higher in athletes than non-athletes and this is particularly so at the sites of the skeleton being exercised most. (On the other hand, bone density falls in hospital patients after prolonged bed rest and in astronauts exposed to a gravity-free environment for long periods.) Weight bearing exercise is therefore important in maintaining bone density. Some calcium may be lost in sweat production but this is small compared with the positive effect that physical activity has on bone mass. Calcium losses in sweat can easily be made up by ensuring an adequate, regular intake of dietary calcium.

Calcium in the Diet

The positive effects of exercise on bone health can be wiped out if calcium intake is regularly low. A reduction in bone mass and bone density can result in an increased risk of stress fractures and can also inhibit proper muscle functioning. Under-consumption of calcium can also increase the risk of developing osteo-porosis in later life. The consequences of not eating enough calcium do not apply only to females, although the long-term problems are less severe for males.

Dairy products are the most effective source of calcium. Unfortunately fear of fat in the diet has led many athletes, mistakenly, to cut out dairy foods such as milk and cheese from their diet. In fact, the fat-reduced milks such as semi-skimmed and skimmed milk actually contain slightly more calcium than full fat milks. This is because the majority of the minerals and vitamins are found in the non-fat part of milk (with, of course the exception of the fat-soluble vitamins). Calcium in vegetables and high-fibre foods may not be as easily absorbed as calcium in milk.

Adequate intakes of calcium, based on the Reference Nutrient Intake (RNI) are import-ant to ensure a high peak bone mass is achieved by young adulthood. Such intakes are also needed throughout adult life to help to slow the rate of bone loss and thus reduce the risk of osteoporosis developing. Athletes who restrict food intake to maintain low body weights may be at particular risk if their diet is habitually low in calcium.

Good Sources of Calcium in the Diet

Dairy Produce

Food	Amount of Calcium
One pint of whole milk	673mg
One pint of semi-skimmed milk	702mg
One pint of skimmed milk	702mg
Matchbox-size piece of Cheddar cheese (40g)	288mg
Matchbox-size piece low fat Cheddar cheese (40g)	336mg
One serving of cottage cheese (4oz/100g)	73mg
One pot of fruit yoghurt (5oz/150g)	225mg

Cereals

Food	Amount of Calcium
Two large slices white or brown	80mg
Two large slices wholemeal bread	39mg

Fish

Food	Amount of Calcium
One can of sardines in tomato sauce including bones (100g)	460mg

Vegetables and Pulses

Food	Amount of Calcium
Three 'spears' of broccoli (150g)	50mg
Quarter of a bunch of watercress	34mg
Two tablespoons (90g) of cooked spinach	144mg
One can of baked beans in tomato sauce (225g)	120mg
Average serving of tofu (bean curd)	306mg

Nuts

Food	Amount of Calcium
One bag of plain peanuts (100g)	60mg
One tablespoon of sesame seeds	80mg

Fruit

Food	Amount of Calcium
Twelve ready to eat dried apricots	73mg
One large orange	50mg

Ice-cream

Food	Amount of Calcium
One scoop dairy ice-cream	78mg

Practical Ways to Increase Calcium Intake

The RNI for calcium for men and women is 700mg a day. If low fat milk and dairy products are consumed on a daily basis this intake can be met, but many athletes struggle to achieve it. The body absorbs calcium from milk and dairy foods better than the calcium from many vegetable sources. Excess protein intake can increase the amount of calcium lost in the urine but foods that contain a high percentage of calcium as well as protein (such as milk and dairy foods) seem to prevent such calcium losses. Simple steps can be taken to increase the calcium content of your diet.

Eat milk or yoghurt with breakfast cereal as this will help to increase the absorption of calcium from the cereal. Add grated reduced fat cheese to salads and soup and sprinkle sesame or sunflower seeds on salads and cooked vegetables. Top home-made pizzas with reduced fat cheese.

Use yoghurt based dressings on salads and top jacket potatoes with plain yoghurt and chives and have one snack of yoghurt, dried apricots or oranges a day. Make milkshakes or smoothies with low fat milk, yoghurt and fruit.

Include dark green vegetables in the diet on a regular basis. Experiment with tofu in stir-fries and salads. Use baked beans more often, either as a quick meal on toast or as a vegetable. Use condensed canned soups and make them up with milk rather than water (if appropriate). Mash up a can of salmon or sardines, including the bones (which contain the calcium), with lemon juice for sandwich fillings.

Make custard with low fat milk to have with fruit, alone or as a frozen dessert and make porridge with milk. Finally, have a milky drink before bed – and that includes hot chocolate.

Iron

Iron is found in haemoglobin in the red blood cells, in myoglobin in the muscle cell and in some of the oxidative enzymes in the mitochondria (the energy producing factories in the cells). A shortage of iron will therefore have a serious effect on energy metabolism. A deficiency of iron is accompanied by common symptoms such as chronic fatigue, susceptibility to stress, increased susceptibility to infections and decreased cognitive performance. Sub-optimal iron status is one of the most common nutritional problems found in the general community and the athletic population group seems to be no exception.

The Vulnerable Athlete

Prolonged hard training has been shown to increase the rate of iron metabolism and decrease iron status. Athletes tend to lose iron through gastro-intestinal bleeding to a greater extent than non-athletes do. Endurance runners seem more prone to this than other athletes, although why this should be is uncertain. Regular use of painkillers such as aspirin may be a contributing factor. Constant striking of the foot during running may cause some bleeding (foot strike haemolysis) which is not a problem for most athletes but could be a problem for endurance runners. Losses of iron in sweat are small and although they may not be sufficient alone to cause iron depletion, they may be a contributing factor. The most likely causes of poor iron status in athletes are the same as those for the general public: poor diet and iron losses during menstruation in women.

Iron Status and Performance

Iron depletion (identified by reduced serum ferritin levels) is not associated with a drop in exercise performance. Iron deficiency is defined as when red blood cell formation is impaired. If red blood cells are not being formed, haemoglobin levels begin to fall towards the lower end of the acceptable range. Again, exercise performance does not appear

<table>
<tr><td>

Possible Causes of Iron Deficiency

- Bleeding in the gastro-intestinal tract.
- Losses in sweat.
- Using up iron stores to make more red blood cells.
- Heavy, regular menstruation in women.
- Poor intake of iron – particularly if red meat is avoided.
- Poor protein intakes.
- Restricted energy intakes.
- Excessive consumption of tea and coffee.

</td></tr>
</table>

does have a negative effect on performance. Iron supplements will correct the iron deficiency anaemia and restore performance levels. However taking iron supplements when there is no iron deficiency anaemia present, even if iron depletion or non-anaemic iron deficiency are present, will not have any effect on performance.

When athletes follow a hard training programme, one of the responses to the training load is an increase in plasma volume. The blood therefore has a greater volume. Although the number of red blood cells and therefore the amount of haemoglobin remains the same, it appears to be less because it is diluted by the increased volume. The concentration of haemoglobin is lower but the ability

to be affected at this stage. However, if this situation is allowed to continue, eventually iron deficiency anaemia will develop and this

---

Good Sources of Iron in the Diet

Animal Sources

Food	Amount of Iron
Two slices of liver (100g)	9mg
One whole pig's kidney (140g)	9mg
One portion of black pudding (75g)	15mg
One serving of lean beef steak (8oz/225g)	6mg
One serving of lean minced beef (4oz/100g)	2.7mg
Two thick slices of corned beef	2.9mg
Pâté, a low fat slice on bread (40g)	2.5mg
One chicken breast	0.65mg
One chicken quarter	2.0mg
One small can of tuna in brine	1.0mg
One large fillet of white fish	0.5mg
Six cockles	6.2mg
Six mussels	3.2mg
One size 3 egg	1.1mg

Cereals

Food	Amount of Iron
Two slices of white bread	1.0mg
Two slices of wholemeal bread	1.9mg
Two Weetabix	3.0mg

Food	Amount of Iron
One serving of Bran Flakes (40g)	8.0mg
Two Shredded Wheat	1.8mg
Three tablespoons muesli (45g)	2.6mg

Vegetables and Pulses

Food	Amount of Iron
Average portion of spinach	1.7mg
Large portion of cabbage	0.7mg
Large portion of peas	1.4mg
One can of baked beans in tomato sauce (225g)	3.2mg
An average portion of tofu (bean curd)	0.7mg

Nuts

Food	Amount of Iron
One bag of cashew nuts (25g)	1.6mg
One tablespoon of sesame seeds	1.1mg

Fruit

Food	Amount of Iron
Twelve ready to eat dried apricots	3.4mg
Six dried dates	1.0mg
Two tablespoons of raisins	0.8mg

to carry oxygen around the body is not reduced. This is often called 'sports anaemia', an unfortunate misnomer as it does not mean there is a lack of iron in the diet nor that an iron supplement is needed.

Iron in the Diet

There are two types of iron in the diet, haem and non-haem iron. Haem iron is found in meat and meat products (particularly offal, liver and kidney, as well as red meat) and non-haem iron is found in cereals, vegetables, peas, beans and lentils and fruits. Haem iron is well absorbed by the body, with up to 20 to 40 per cent being taken up whereas only 5 to 20 per cent of iron from vegetable sources, egg and milk is absorbed. Overall, for adults eating a mixed diet including meat and fish, absorption is assumed to be about 15 per cent. As with milk and dairy foods, many athletes avoid meat because of the perceived fat content. In fact the fat content of lean red meat has fallen by one third on average over the last twenty years by a combination of breeding, feed changes and modern butchery techniques. There are a variety of good and valid reasons why an athlete might choose not to eat meat but fat content is not one of them.

Practical Ways to Increase Iron Intakes

The RNI for iron for women (aged 11 to 50 years) is 14.8mg a day and for adult men it is 8.7mg a day. The RNI for women is higher to make up for iron losses due to menstruation.

The following are simple ways in which you can ensure that your intake of iron is sufficient.

- If appropriate, eat red meat, pork or poultry three or four times a week.
- Choose breakfast cereals that are fortified with iron (information on iron content will be given on the packet).
- Ensure vitamin C rich foods and drinks are eaten with foods containing iron, particu-

larly non-haem iron foods, as vitamin C helps the absorption of iron. For example, drink a glass of orange juice along with cereal at breakfast, chose egg and tomato or watercress sandwiches or drink grapefruit juice as a starter before the meat course. (*See* Chapter 1 for good sources of vitamin C.)

- Avoid drinking tea and coffee with meals as the tannin in these drinks can reduce iron absorption.
- Avoid adding extra bran to food and choose foods containing natural fibre instead. Excessive bran intakes can reduce iron absorption.
- Absorption of iron from vegetables and cereals can be improved by eating a source of animal protein such as red meat at the same meal.
- The following combinations can help maximise iron absorption: baked beans on toast, dried apricots added to meat dishes (if appropriate), dried fruit added to breakfast cereals, beans and meat (for example chilli con carne), lentil soup and bread, stir-fried meats with added broccoli sprigs and peppers, mixed beans added to salad.

Non-meat eaters should ensure that their diet contains some of the following on a daily basis:

- Wholegrain cereals and flours such as wheat, rye, millet and oatmeal.
- Nuts, for example almonds, Brazil nuts, cashews and hazelnuts.
- Green vegetables, for example cabbage, watercress, spinach, broccoli and parsley.
- Pulses, for example soya beans, chickpeas, baked beans and lentils.
- Dried fruit, for example apricots, prunes, raisins.
- Seeds, for example pumpkin, sesame and sunflower seeds.

Other useful food items include brewer's yeast, curry powder, textured vegetable protein, soya flour, black treacle, molasses, chocolate, cocoa and ginger.

Salt

General dietary guidelines for health encourage a reduction in salt intake because of the possible link between regular high intakes and the development of high blood pressure. This is another example where guidelines for the general public may not be appropriate for the exercising and sporting population. Salt lost through sweating must be replaced and intakes for athletes should be higher than the general recommendations.

Sweat composition varies considerably between individuals. It also varies with time during a period of exercise and is influenced by the state of acclimatisation. Concerns over the possible adverse effects of a high salt intake have resulted in some athletes restricting their intakes. However raising intakes above the general public recommendations could benefit athletes as long as overall fluid intake is good and kidneys are functioning well. This is best achieved by adding some salt to meals when sweat losses have been high.

Other Minerals

Calcium and iron present specific problems because the best dietary sources are sometimes foods that are excluded from the diet for a variety of reasons, some of which are valid but others which are based on misconceptions and misinformation. Other minerals may be lost from the body during exercise and training but these will normally be replenished by following a diet that contains a wide range of foods in sufficient quantity to meet overall energy requirements.

Athletes who have poor diets or who are

Upper Safe Levels for Long Term Use of Daily Mineral Supplements	
Mineral	Quantity
Calcium	1,500mg
Phosphorus	1,500mg
Magnesium	300mg
Iron	15mg
Zinc	15mg
Copper	5mg
Selenium	200µg
Iodine	500µg
Manganese	15mg
Chromium	200µg
Molybdenum	200µg

(Source: Council for Responsible Nutrition, an association of leading suppliers of food supplements and the European Federation of Associations of Health Product Manufacturers which represents specialist health product manufacturers in Europe.)

These intakes of vitamins are in addition to the amounts gained from the diet. The upper safe level for supplementation is an indication to consumers of levels of consumption that it would be unwise to exceed. It is not a definition of levels that could be advocated to promote general health.

maintaining a low food intake in order to reduce body weight/body fat should be advised to take a multivitamin/mineral supplement on a regular basis. This should contain no more than the Recommended Daily Amount (RDA) of each vitamin or mineral. Large doses of minerals can interact with each other, affecting absorption and function, and are not recommended.

WATER

Keeping well-hydrated or at least minimizing dehydration is vital both in training and

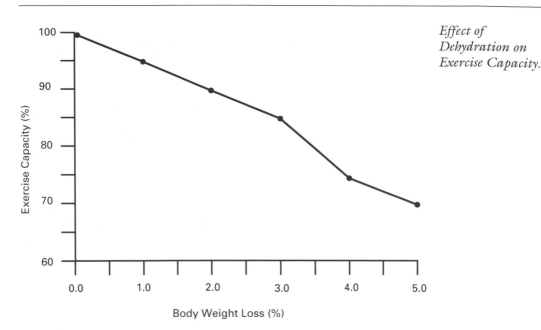

Effect of Dehydration on Exercise Capacity.

competition. This applies just as much to the strength and speed athlete as to the endurance athlete, to the individual athlete as to the team player. If a sprinter starts a race dehydrated, this can slow the initial reaction-response to the gun and the actual start of movement. In team sports, mental function is vital for reading the game, decision making, anticipation and skill delivery. Keeping well hydrated should be the goal of all athletes if both physical and mental performance are to be optimized. A loss of 2 per cent of body weight through sweat loss can reduce aerobic capacity by up to 20 per cent. A loss of 5 per cent of body weight can reduce it by as much as 30 per cent

A typical sedentary individual in the UK loses between 2 and 3 litres of water from the body every day. In very hot conditions, the water loss may increase to between 4 and 10 litres per day. During exercise the fluid losses can vary enormously depending on a variety of factors (*see* Chapter 2). Evaporation of sweat can exceed 1.5 litres per hour and it

has been estimated that Tour de France cyclists may sweat out as much as 2.5 litres per hour. Fluid losses must be minimized and the losses that do occur must be replaced quickly.

Dehydration not only has a detrimental effect on performance but can also become a health risk as the level of dehydration increases.

Can the Body Adjust to Dehydration?

In time the body adjusts to cope with the need to increase fluid intake to compensate for the fluid losses through sweating. A new balance between output and intake is established. This new balance involves an increase in fluid intake with no increase in urine output – the extra fluid is all lost in sweat.

A person travelling to a hot climate will be dehydrated for the first few days until this re-adjustment has taken place. Thirst itself is not a sufficiently powerful stimulus to ensure sufficient intake of liquids in this early period of exposure and a conscious effort to drink

A runner passing a water station during the London Marathon.

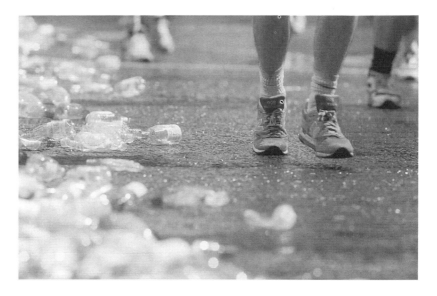

must be made, even when there are no thirst feelings. Thirst does not become apparent until a significant level of dehydration has occurred.

Long-haul flights can lead to a state of dehydration before training, competition or indeed the holiday has even begun. The low water vapour pressure in the cabin causes an increase in fluid loss from the body. Very few travellers drink enough while flying to compensate for these losses. Tea, coffee and alcohol all stimulate urine output and make any dehydration even worse. The fact that many people urinate very little for the first few days in the heat is a clear indication of dehydration.

The body can only maintain maximum performance if dehydration is limited as much as possible and this is only achieved by working at maintaining fluid intake. Drinking sufficient fluids to maintain water balance, particularly in conditions where fluid losses are increased, does not happen without effort, and in some cases considerable effort. The body cannot be trained to get used to dehydration.

The Mechanics of Fluid Replacement

It is important that fluids are made available to the body as quickly as possible. The two limiting factors are how quickly the fluid leaves the stomach and how quickly it is absorbed in the small intestine. Factors that affect stomach emptying include caloric density, osmolality (a measure for the osmotic pressure which a solution exerts across a biological membrane, in general determined by the number of particles in solution), volume, acidity, temperature and sodium concentration. Caloric density has the greatest impact: the greater number of calories the slower the emptying time. Increase in osmolality of the stomach contents tends to delay emptying although there is evidence that the use of glucose polymers instead of glucose allows a greater concentration of glucose without reducing the rate of emptying.

In the small intestine, the presence of glucose stimulates sodium uptake from the small intestine and this greatly increases fluid absorption. The active transport of glucose and sodium creates an osmotic gradient which

Summary of Factors Affecting Stomach Emptying	
Factor	*Effect on Stomach Emptying*
Volume	High volume speeds up emptying.
Fat	High fat content slows emptying.
Osmolality	Hypertonic solutions slow emptying.
pH	Low pH (more acid) slows emptying.
Calorie density	High calorie density slows emptying.
Carbohydrate concentration	> 6 to 8 per cent slows emptying.
Carbohydrate type	No effect.
Exercise type	No effect.
Exercise level	0 to 70 per cent VO2max no effect; > 75 per cent VO2max slows emptying.
Dehydration	Slows emptying during exercise.

draws water across the gut wall. Other carbohydrates such as sucrose or glucose polymers can be substituted for glucose without impairing glucose or water uptake.

Sports Drinks

Carbohydrate Content

Glucose, glucose polymers or maltodextrin or sucrose and fructose are all used in sports drinks and they all empty from the stomach at similar rates, so the type of carbohydrate ingested does not have a major influence on gastric emptying time. Glucose, glucose polymers and sucrose all stimulate absorption in the small intestine but fructose absorption is slower and therefore does not stimulate as much fluid absorption.

It is now known that drinks containing 6 to 8 per cent glucose or sucrose are absorbed into

the body more rapidly than water and, unlike water, they provide some energy (for the working muscles). A slightly higher concentration of carbohydrate can be used if the carbohydrate source is a glucose polymer or maltodextrin. Both a single glucose unit or molecule or several units of glucose joined together to make a polymer of glucose will each contribute one particle. A greater amount of carbohydrate (energy) can be delivered by a glucose polymer drink without compromising the rate of stomach emptying. Some sports drinks contain lower concentrations of carbohydrate (1 to 3 per cent), as do the oral rehydration solutions for use when suffering from diarrhoea, but they will obviously not supply as much energy to the muscles.

What Does 'Isotonic' Mean?

The isotonicity has considerable bearing on the effectiveness of the drink. An isotonic drink has the same number of dissolved particles as are found in plasma (about 290mosmol per kg). The dissolved particles will be electrolytes and carbohydrates such as the simple sugars or glucose polymers. Isotonic drinks promote a high carbohydrate and fluid delivery.

A less concentrated drink has a lower osmolality (hypotonic) and promotes water uptake but usually supplies less carbohydrate. Drinks which are hypertonic have a greater osmolality. They contain a greater concentration of carbohydrate and will therefore deliver more energy. However this will slow up the gastric emptying and compromise fluid replacement. Fatigue is likely to occur due to depletion of glycogen or to dehydration.

In the ideal situation, the type of drink taken during exercise should reflect this. Where rehydration is the priority, an isotonic drink containing no more than 8 per cent carbohydrate should be used. Where provision of fuel takes priority over fluid replacement, a more concentrated solution can be used.

Electrolytes
Sodium is added to sports drinks to stimulate the absorption of water in the small intestine. Although some electrolytes are lost from the body through sweating, a much greater proportion of fluid is also lost, so that the net effect is an increase in electrolyte concentration in the plasma. Fluid replacement rather than electrolyte replacement is the primary need. However, sodium replacement promotes water absorption, and the supply of other electrolytes in quantities not exceeding quantities lost in sweat does not appear to influence fluid uptake negatively, nor affect blood electrolyte levels.

Replacement of water in the post-exercise period can be crucial but drinking plain water is not the most effective way to achieve this. Water alone causes changes in the plasma sodium concentration and in plasma osmolality. These changes reduce the stimulus to drink (the thirst mechanism) and stimulate urine output, both of which delay the rehydration process. Most fizzy soft drinks such as colas contain virtually no sodium so these are also not ideal.

The oral rehydration solutions (ORS) such as Dioralyte and Rehidrat used in cases of dehydration caused by severe diarrhoea were the drawing board for the composition of many sports drinks. ORS contain 60 to 90mmol of sodium per litre, essentially more than is lost in sweat. A high sodium content tends to make drinks unpalatable, although taste for salt does change when an individual is dehydrated and body temperature is elevated.

However it is important that drinks designed to be drunk during and after exercise taste pleasant as this encourages drinking. An ideal formulation is no longer ideal if nobody drinks it. Sports drinks tend to contain 10 to 25mmol sodium per litre – a compromise between what is desirable physiologically and what is palatable.

Other Electrolytes
Although there seems no doubt about the need for sodium, there has been some debate about the value of adding other electrolytes. Potassium is found in intracellular fluid and it has been suggested that its addition to sports drinks might help in the rehydration process. The water lost as sweat comes from the plasma, extracellular fluid and the intracellular fluid, which supports the theory that addition of potassium might help water retention in the intracellular fluid.

Most sports drinks do contain other electrolytes in addition to sodium, often in concentrations similar to those estimated to be present in sweat. It is generally considered that such losses can be made up easily by the normal food intake. As far as adverse effects of adding other electrolytes are concerned, there appear to be no reported cases and with the widespread usage of such drinks one would, by this time, have expected any significant problems to have come to light.

Other Ingredients
A quick glance at the ingredient declaration of sports drinks on pack will show a wide variety of extra ingredients over and above carbohydrate and sodium. These include ingredients added for palatability and consumer appeal (flavourings, colours, artificial sweeteners) and additives to help in processing and to produce a stable safe product (stabilisers, preservatives and acidity regulators). Many commercially available products also contain added vitamins although there is no evidence to suggest they play a role in rehydration or need to be supplied in any way other than from the normal diet.

Sports drinks are often used as a vehicle for the addition of ingredients that might be perceived to have a performance enhancing effect. For example, caffeine, taurine, co-enzyme Q10 and many others have been used. However the addition of ingredients that should be taken in controlled dosages or amounts to a drink that will by its very nature be consumed in variable amounts is debatable.

Some products are carbonated and there is some evidence that gastric emptying is hastened if drinks are carbonated. Highly carbonated drinks, however, are likely to cause gastro-intestinal distress.

What is the Ideal Sports Drink?

The ideal sports rehydration drink must contain carbohydrate, sodium and of course water. It must be hypotonic or isotonic and palatable and easy to use. The addition of other electrolytes may have a small advantage in helping to replace sweat losses, although the bulk of this replacement will come from food intake. Sweat rates are very individual and depend on a range of factors. There is obviously no single drink that is ideal in all situations or, indeed, for all individuals. Commercial sports drinks are a reasonable compromise. They help to rehydrate the body quickly and effectively and at the same time provide extra energy to supplement the body's limited carbohydrate stores.

Maintaining Hydration

A variety of factors affect fluid intake during exercise and sport, some relating to the individual athlete and others to the sport itself. In many situations fluid intake can be improved by a better understanding of the importance of fluid in preventing dehydration by athletes, coaches, teachers and National and International Governing Bodies. Certainly the misconception that it is possible to adapt to exercising in a dehydrated state must be corrected.

The following factors often influence decisions regarding fluid intake.

Lack of thirst. Even though the athlete is becoming dehydrated, there is no prompt to drink.

Visible sweat losses. These may remind the athlete to drink but possibly not in sufficient quantities. Sweat losses are not always obvious, for example in water sports where the body is already wet or in cycling where the skin is dried quickly by the wind.

Availability of fluids. If no fluids are provided at the training venue, the athletes must remember to provide their own drinks and drinks bottles. Coolers provided in the vicinity of the training venue can encourage a better fluid intake.

Opportunity to drink. This is often dependent on others (such as the coach or teacher) or on the particular rules of the sport (the availability of formal breaks or stoppages).

Palatability of the drink. The flavour, taste, mouth-feel and temperature of the drink can affect the amount that is drunk.

Gastro-intestinal discomfort, or the fear of it. This highlights the need to use training

Carbohydrate and Sodium Content of Some Commonly Used Sports Drinks		
Drink	Carbohydrate g/100ml	Sodium mg/100ml
Isostar	7.7	70
Gatorade	6	41
Lucozade Sport	6.4	50
Boots Isotonic	8.6	18
Maxim Electrolyte	7.4	69
High5 Isotonic	7.36	62.7

sessions to find comfort zones and develop individual strategies of what, when and how much should be drunk. The nausea experienced by some athletes could be caused by dehydration itself or the consumption of a drink which is too concentrated.

Call of nature. A fear of needing to urinate during a match or a race can lead to restricted fluid intakes prior to events.

Lack of knowledge. If there is a poor understanding of the need to maintain hydration and the effect dehydration has on both physical and mental performance and ultimately health, athletes are unlikely to work at maintaining hydration status.

Weight issues. Athletes may avoid sports drinks with a calorie value. Dehydration may be deliberately used as a method of weight loss for competition in weight-category sports.

What to Drink

During the day, athletes should enjoy a range of drinks including water (tap, bottled, fizzy or still), fruit juice, squashes, soft drinks, tea and coffee. Diet soft drinks may be appropriate, particularly for those athletes who are restricting their energy intake to lose weight.

Coffee and tea contain caffeine which acts as a diuretic and so stimulates urine production. In the past the advice has been to encourage a reduction in intake or a switch to decaffeinated varieties. It now seems that regular drinkers of caffeine-containing drinks adapt to the caffeine intake and that the diuretic effects become less apparent.

As with food, it is best to include a variety of drinks each day. Prior to, during and immediately after training and competition, a sports drink (commercial or home-made) will in many situations be the first choice drink.

Recipes for Home-Made Isotonic Drinks

50 to 70g glucose or sucrose (ordinary sugar)
1 litre warm water
1 large pinch of salt (1.0 to 1.5g)

Warm a small amount of the water and use to dissolve the glucose and salt. Flavour with low sugar or low calorie squash (not regular squash as this will upset the balance of carbohydrate). Top up to a litre with water. Mix together, cover and keep chilled in the fridge.

500ml unsweetened fruit juice (for example orange, pineapple or grapefruit)
500ml water
1 large pinch of salt (1.0 to 1.5g)

Warm a small amount of the water and use this to dissolve the salt. Add the fruit juice and remaining cold water. Mix together, cover and keep chilled in the fridge.

200 ml squash (any flavour but not low sugar or no added sugar varieties)
800 ml water
1 large pinch of salt (1.0 to 1.5g)

Warm a small amount of the water and use this to dissolve the salt. Add the squash and remaining cold water. Mix together, cover and keep chilled in the fridge.

Make up a new batch of drink every day and throw away any unused drink after 24 hours. Keep water bottles very clean. Sugary drinks attract insects and will provide fertile breeding grounds for bacteria. This is important at all times but especially during warm weather.

The Temperature of the Drink

When training or competing in warm conditions, chilled drinks usually taste better but some athletes like drinks as cold as 5 to 10°C.

87

However tolerance to cold drinks is individual and drinks as cold as this can cause gastro-intestinal upsets in some people.

Cold drinks were believed to empty from the stomach faster than warm drinks but this is no longer thought to be true. Indeed a warm drink (at a temperature which allows it to be drunk quickly) will not delay stomach emptying nor affect the thermo-regulatory mechanism. Such drinks could therefore give a lift to a tiring athlete exercising in a cold climate without affecting performance.

How Much to Drink

For low intensity exercise, such as walking or gently cycling or for exercise lasting no more than thirty minutes, there is probably no requirement to drink. However athletes must start well hydrated and rehydrate afterwards and take account of weather conditions. If it is very warm, even gentle exercise will lead to some sweat loss.

Numerous guidelines are available but, by definition, these are only guidelines. The most well known advice is the American College of Sports Medicine (ACSM) recommendation on exercise and fluid replacement. It is recommended that individuals drink about 500ml of fluid about two hours before exercise to promote adequate hydration and allow time for excretion of excess ingested water. During intense exercise lasting longer than one hour, it is recommended that 600 to 1,200ml per hour of solutions containing 4 to 8 per cent carbohydrate are drunk. Although the ACSM did not give a specific recommendation for fluid intake following exercise, there was agreement that intake should be based on pre and post-exercise body weight and that enough fluid should be drunk to restore body weight, taking into account obligatory urine losses.

With practice, athletes can often manage to drink more fluid before the start of a training session or competition than the ACSM guidelines. This is particularly important if large sweat losses are anticipated. Drinking 500ml in the last hour is not uncommon nor indeed is drinking 300 to 500ml in the last fifteen minutes before exercise, although it is important to urinate just before the start of training.

Athletes ideally need to know their own requirements rather than just applying guidelines. Two athletes of the same height and weight taking part in the same training sessions will not necessarily sweat at the same rates. Individual sweat losses can be estimated quite simply and this practice should be encouraged. Knowing his or her own likely sweat losses in different situations (hard or light training sessions, hot or cold days, high or low humidity) can help an athlete to anticipate fluid losses and therefore estimate how much to drink to minimize or avoid dehydration.

Sweat loss can be estimated by weighing before and after the training session. Weighing should be done naked or, if this is not practical, wearing the minimum of dry clothing with the body towelled down. The aim is to make the weighing conditions at both times as similar as possible, so sweaty clothing should not be worn for the post-training weighing. If possible, fluid intake should match weight loss so that weight after training is the same or even slightly higher than the weight before training (to cover continuing fluid losses after the session). Reliable scales should be used, ideally weighing to the nearest 100g.

The difference in weight before and after training is primarily due to the fluid losses that have not been made up or prevented by fluid intake during the training session. A loss of 1kg is equivalent to a litre of fluid that has been lost but not replaced. By measuring the amount of fluid drunk during the session, the total sweat loss can be calculated.

Total sweat loss = weight before training

minus weight after training plus weight or volume of fluid drunk.

To cover the continuing loss of sweat after exercise finishes and the urine losses that persist even in the dehydrated state, it is now generally recommended that for every 1kg loss, an intake of 1.5 litres is needed.

Knowing sweat losses in different situations can help an athlete to build up a fluid strategy. This can be particularly helpful for athletes who compete away from home. In these situations, routine becomes disrupted and fluid intake may be less than usual, which is hardly good preparation for competition.

Monitoring body weight first thing in the morning can be a way of identifying chronic dehydration. However progressive weight loss may also be due to insufficient calorie intake. A simple pinch test can also be used as a rough guide. The skin on the back of the hand is pinched. In a well-hydrated athlete, the skin snaps back at once but if the skin stays pinched for several seconds, fluids need to be taken on board.

There are numerous practical ways to ensure adequate hydration is maintained, but the overall message is to maintain fluid intake at all times, not just around training and competitions. It is important to include a variety of different drinks and to use sports drinks when this is appropriate for the type and duration of the training session or competition.

Athletes should begin all training sessions and competitions fully hydrated. This will require adequate fluid intake throughout every day with particular attention to ensuring optimal rehydration after any previous training session.

Aim to drink early in the training session and then at regular intervals. Starting with small regular intakes, it will not be long before 150 to 250ml every fifteen minutes can be drunk comfortably. The stomach empties at around 1,000 to 1,200ml per hour – the greater the volume, the faster it empties. It takes no more than ten to twenty minutes for fluids to travel from the gut to the skin for sweating, hence the need to start drinking sooner rather than later. Thirst is an unreliable indicator of fluid requirement. Athletes need to drink fluids before the stimulation of the thirst mechanism kicks in. Waiting until you feel thirsty will invariably be too late to be of any benefit.

The 'pee test' is a simple method of detecting the level of hydration or dehydration. Passing urine which is pale in colour (especially by late evening) frequently and in reasonable volumes are signs of being hydrated. Small volumes of dark urine, passed infrequently or failure to urinate for long periods of time are all warning signs of dehydration. (Regular use of multivitamin supplements can make urine yellower in colour. This should be considered the baseline colour and any further darkening from this could indicate dehydration.)

At the first sign of dehydration, fluids should be consumed and continued until urination returns to normal. Isotonic or hypotonic sports drinks or the oral rehydration fluids would be sensible choices.

Laminated pee charts and A4 posters can be bought from the Sports Nutrition Interest

What is a 2 Per Cent Body Loss?			
Pre-Exercise Body Weight		*Weight Loss After Exercise Equivalent to 2 Per Cent of Body Weight*	
kg	*lb*	*kg*	*lb*
50	110	1.0	2.2
60	132	1.2	2.6
70	154	1.4	3.0
80	176	1.6	3.5
90	198	1.8	4.0
100	220	2.0	4.4

Group of the British Dietetic Association (*see* Appendix IV for address).

Where possible, training sessions should be used to experiment with different drinks to discover which is most palatable. It is easier to drink a large volume of a palatable drink than one that does not taste so good. Training sessions should also be used to build up and get accustomed to the required fluid intakes.

Fluid intake should be started as soon as possible into the training session. (This may be limited by the coach or teacher, in which case the key is to begin at the first opportunity.) The aim is to prevent dehydration rather than trying to reverse it. Likely sweat loss during exercise should be anticipated (using information from the weighing exercises) and efforts made to drink as much as possible to minimize the loss. Choose drinks bottles which are large enough to provide the likely volume needed. In some conditions, two or more bottles may be needed.

In some situations it is difficult to maintain fluid intakes. For example it is possible to carry a fluid bottle during runs of about forty-five minutes, but as the duration of the run gets progressively longer it becomes impractical to carry the amount of fluid needed. It may be necessary to arrange drinks along the route, to devise a run that laps round home where empty bottles can be exchanged for full ones or to arrange for a minder to cycle alongside with supplies.

Some athletes only drink during competition, never in training. This should be discouraged. Drinking during training ensures the athlete is getting maximum out of the sessions and not fatiguing early and also that the athlete is getting used to drinking and the sensation of fluid in the stomach while exercising. This will obviously be of benefit when it comes to competitions.

Large volumes of fluid empty from the stomach more rapidly than small volumes but it is important to build up fluid intake slowly. Athletes must train themselves to ingest larger volumes of fluid more frequently.

The rehydration process should be continued as soon as possible after exercise. This is particularly important if there is a further training session or competition later in the day.

Athletes should get into the habit of keeping a bottle of water with them at all times and taking regular water breaks throughout the day (for example by keeping a bottle of water in the car and on the desk at work, a jug of water in the fridge and a bottle of water by the bed). It is surprising how the sips taken can mount up through the day. Plain water can be livened up with a slice of lemon or a sprig of mint.

Athletes should be encouraged to drink water at key points throughout the day: on waking, at mealtimes, arriving at work, getting home after work, during coffee breaks and at bedtime. Fluid routines should be maintained even when daily routine is changed. This may be particularly relevant when travelling. It is prudent to keep a check on the weather and to plan fluid intake accordingly.

Ideally, clothing should be light and airy. Sweat evaporation can be impaired by inappropriate clothing such as multiple layer and protective clothing. It is best to keep wearing a wet shirt rather than changing into a dry one during a break in training or competition. A wet shirt cools the body down more effectively than a dry one.

Salt tablets should be avoided as they are too concentrated and need a lot of water to be utilized. They can also irritate the gut and cause diarrhoea and vomiting. Care is needed if using carbohydrate gels because energy levels are dipping. Taken with too little water they can actually pull water into the gut and lower blood volume, which is the exact opposite of what is needed.

Alcohol should not be drunk until full hydration status has been restored by drinking sports drinks, fruit juice, squashes or soft drinks. Once copious amounts of urine are being produced, it is okay to drink alcohol. The same applies to caffeine containing drinks such as tea, coffee, colas and certain energy drinks. Alcohol and caffeine are both diuretics and will dehydrate rather than rehydrate.

Care of Teeth

Dental decay is caused by dental plaque (a thin layer of bacteria sticking to the teeth) converting dietary sugars into acids which then attack the teeth. Anything that contains sugars will have the ability to contribute to dental decay. Dental erosion is a different problem and occurs when acids from the diet (or regurgitated from the stomach) dissolve the tooth surface. Dietary acids are found in fruits (particularly citrus fruits), fruit juices, fruit based and fizzy soft drinks, pickled foods or foods containing vinegar and sports drinks.

Dentists accept that rehydration is vital for athletes and that sports drinks play an important part, indeed the British Dental Association has produced guidelines to help athletes minimize the risks of dental decay and dental erosion.

- Effective daily brushing and flossing to reduce the risk of dental decay.
- Drink sports drinks quickly, preferably with a straw.
- Avoid sipping, holding or swishing drinks in the mouth.
- Drink cool drinks to help reduce erosion.
- Rinse the mouth after acidic drinks rather than brushing. Brushing is more likely to wear away the teeth.
- Avoid excessive use of acidic drinks during the day and limit use of sports drinks to before, during and after exercise.

- Chewing sugar free gum can help to protect against dental erosion by increasing saliva production, although this is only recommended after exercise. Gum should never be chewed while exercising.
- Have regular check-ups with a dentist and hygienist.

A Final Warning

It is important that athletes are aware of the key signs of dehydration, not just in themselves but in others. This also applies to coaches and teachers. Acute signs (which may occur in as little as one hour) include nausea, poor concentration, flushed skin and light-headedness. Over a period of hours or a day, chronic signs to look out for are loss of appetite, dark yellow urine, little or no urination and muscle cramps.

ALCOHOL

Alcohol consumption plays a prominent part in the social side of many sports and is the most widely used drug amongst athletes. Yet it can affect sporting performance, not in an enhancing way as some athletes believe, but in a detrimental way. Alcohol has been alleged to alter energy metabolism, improve physiological processes and modify other factors.

Energy Metabolism

Although alcohol contains a relatively large number of calories and its metabolic pathways in the body are short, the available evidence suggests that it is not used to any significant extent as a source of fuel during exercise.

First the major sources of energy for exercise are carbohydrates and fats – and these are in ample supply in most individuals. Second,

Typical Effects of Increasing Blood Alcohol Level		
Number of Drinks in Two Hours	Blood Alcohol Level (mg per litre)	Typical Effects
2 to 3	20 to 40	Reduced tension, relaxed state
4 to 5	60 to 90	Impaired judgement, euphoria, impaired fine motor skills and co-ordination
6 to 9	110 to 160	Slurred speech, impaired gross motor co-ordination, staggering gait
9 to 12	180 to 250	Loss of control of voluntary activity, erratic behaviour, impaired vision
13 to 18	270 to 390	Stupor, total loss of co-ordination
more than 19	more than 400	Coma, death

though the by-products formed when alcohol is broken down and released by the liver may find their way into muscles, they appear to be of little importance as a fuel source. Thirdly, using alcohol would be a very uneconomical way of fuelling exercise as the amount of oxygen needed to release the energy from alcohol is greater than for an equivalent amount of carbohydrate or fat. Lastly, the rate that the liver metabolizes alcohol is too slow to make it a useful energy source, particularly for those involved in high intensity exercise when energy must be supplied very rapidly.

Physiological Processes

Alcohol in small amounts (one or two drinks) does not improve or impair physiological processes associated with maximal aerobic exercise such as VO2max and maximal heart rate. Nor does it seem to affect strength and local muscular endurance. However alcohol may interfere with glucose metabolism during exercise. In endurance exercise, such as marathons, this could lead to low blood glucose levels or hypoglycaemia or depletion of glycogen stores in the muscles. In other words fuel would start to run out earlier with a subsequent drop in performance. It is a myth that alcohol can be sweated out. Only a tiny amount is detected in sweat: the vast majority of the alcohol consumed is metabolized in the liver.

Other Factors

There is ample evidence that alcohol adversely affects psychomotor performance, such as reaction time, balance, concentration, hand-eye co-ordination and visual perception. Alcohol ingestion may also impair body temperature regulation during prolonged exercise in a cold environment. There is also the possibility that drinking alcohol before exercise may be the prelude to an accident which could cause injury or even death.

The use of alcohol in competition is formally prohibited in the sport of modern pentathlon (where events include fencing, shooting and horse riding as well as swimming and running). Testing for alcohol may be requested by any National Governing Body and a positive test could lead to sanctions.

Alcohol has been used to help reduce pain, improve confidence and to help to override other psychological barriers to performance. It may also be used to stimulate the cardio-vascular system or to reduce tremor in precision sports such as archery, rifle shooting and darts.

The effects of alcohol are very much dose related. Tests of reaction time, strength, power and cardiovascular performance are not adversely affected if only one or two alcoholic drinks have been consumed the night before. On the other hand, heavy drinking may impair performance on the following day due to the effects of a hangover. An alcohol hangover is caused by alcohol toxicity, dehydration and the toxic effects of the congeners in alcoholic drinks. It is commonly characterized by a depressed mood, headache and hypersensitivity to outside stimuli. As a result an athlete with a hangover may not perform at his or her best.

Alcohol can slow injury recovery as it causes the blood vessels to the skin, arms and legs to open up. The increased blood supply makes any injury bleed and swell even more and can therefore slow the recovery process.

The consumption of alcohol, usually in the form of beer, is a common practice after many sporting events. Although the alcohol may produce feelings of relaxation, the athlete is more prone to possible adverse effects. High intakes of alcohol may prevent athletes from consuming enough carbohydrate to optimize muscle glycogen storage. Beer is also not an ideal drink for rehydration purposes as it has a very low sodium content. After exercise, the stomach of the athlete is usually empty and the body dehydrated so any alcohol is absorbed rapidly and not diluted. This leads to a rapid rise in the level of alcohol in the blood,

---

Practical Advice About Alcohol

Never make alcohol the first drink after exercise but wait to be well hydrated and to have refuelled effectively before drinking alcohol. Avoid alcohol for at least 24 hours after exercise if a soft tissue injury or bruising has occurred. Avoid alcohol in the 24 hours leading up to a competition, match or race.

The Health Education Authority and other medical experts suggest men should drink less than 21 units per week and women less than 14 units a week to avoid damaging health. Drinks should be spread through the week, binge drinking should be avoided and there should be two or three alcohol-free days each week.

One unit of alcohol equals:

- One single pub measure of spirits.
- One single pub measure of liqueur.
- One small glass of sherry or fortified wine.
- One small glass of wine.

- Half a pint of lager, beer or cider (regular strength).

Extend alcoholic drinks by adding soda water, low caloric mixers or mineral water. Spritzers are now very socially acceptable drinks. Drink slowly and avoid getting into a pattern of buying rounds which might encourage drinking more quickly and a greater number of drinks than you are comfortable with. Alternate low or no alcohol drinks (mineral water, fruit juice, low calorie mixers or soft drinks) with alcoholic drinks.

Exercise care when drinking at home. Measures poured at home are invariably much larger than pub measures. Finish a drink before allowing it to be topped up, for example when drinking wine in restaurants.

Drinking on an empty stomach speeds up alcohol absorption so always eat first or alternatively drink only with meals.

which could have serious implications if the athlete intends to drive home.

Chronic consumption of large amounts of alcohol carry both health and social problems as well as obvious effects on performance. There may be a resulting poor dietary intake, poor lifestyle including inadequate rest and excessive caloric intake from alcohol leading to weight gain. A common problem in seasonal sports is the increase in weight and particularly body fat in the off-season when diet is relaxed and alcohol intake increases while physical activity levels plummet.

PRACTICAL ADVICE

Pulling all this information together and converting it into suitable main meals, light meals and refuelling snacks can be daunting, particularly for the athlete who lacks time and cooking skills.

Time Management

Athletes invariably have very little time to shop, prepare and cook food let alone sit down and eat it. They are often so tired after a hard evening training session they cannot be bothered to start preparing a meal, even though they know they should be refuelling before going to bed.

With planning and organisation, dietary goals can be met and enjoyable well-balanced meals can be produced quickly. Many recipe books give preparation time (active time that needs full attention) and cooking time (passive time when the oven can do the work). For example, a roast dinner does not require much active time but cooking time may be an hour or more. This is not the best choice when time is short but, on the other hand, it may be possible to prepare the food and then leave it to cook while training or resting. A roasted

---

Getting Organized

Keep store-cupboards, fridge and freezer stocked with ingredients, particularly those that can be used to make quick meals (*see* Appendix 1). If you know that there is food readily available you will be less tempted to eat junk food on the way home from training or work.

Keep kitchen utensils and equipment in good order and invest in key timesaving kitchen equipment such as a microwave oven, toaster, pressure cooker and wok.

Plan ahead by cooking meals for the week in one session and then freezing them, or by cooking a double portion and freezing the extra portion. Defrost a meal in the morning ready for reheating in the evening.

When sharing accommodation, take it in turns to prepare the evening meal.

Keep a shopping list handy so you can note items which are about to run out and need to be replaced. The time to add 'baked beans' to the shopping list is when the next to last can is opened.

---

joint of meat will usually provide enough cold meat for a meal the next day, thus saving time and money.

Going Shopping

Making a shopping list is the best way of making sure that only essential items are bought and that money is not squandered on unnecessary goods. It is a good idea to have at least a rough plan of the week's meals and therefore the items that are needed.

Labels on food packaging now give a lot of useful information so that you can tell at a glance how much carbohydrate is present, whether the fat content is high and whether there are any special storage or cooking instructions – in other words if the item is a good buy. Comparing costs of different brands of the same item can take time, but if money is an issue, this will be time well spent. Sell by dates should also be checked so that packets with the longest shelf life can be selected.

Once home with the shopping, it is important to store items promptly and prop erly. New items should be put to the back and older ones brought to the front (this applies to tins and cans as well as to more obviously perishable items such as yoghurts).

Keeping the Cost Down

For athletes with high energy demands, food bills can grow quite large. For others money may be tight for a variety of reasons. In either case, a few simple guidelines may help to make money go further while eating enough to meet the necessary requirements and enjoying it along the way.

If possible, buy all the dry goods and some perishables at the beginning of the week and then buy more perishables for the end of the week a few days later. That way food will not end up being thrown away. This particularly applies to fresh fruit and vegetables.

Check prices at supermarkets and compare them with those charged by the local butcher, greengrocer and market stalls. The super-market may not be the cheapest place to buy meat, fruit and vegetables. Special offers can save money, but only if they fit into the eating plan and will be eaten before the 'best before' date. The same applies to money-off coupons. Buying own brand products whenever possible can help to keep the cost down. Check receipts to see where the money is going and if it is being spent wisely.

Prices are often reduced towards the end of the day, although there are not so many late Saturday afternoon bargains since Sunday trading became legalized. Buying in bulk and sharing with similar minded friends can make a great saving on bills, particularly if it is possible to visit a cash and carry outlet.

It is a good idea to shop on the way home so the time between buying and storing is kept to a minimum in order to maximize shelf life, preserve nutrients and reduce any wastage. This particularly applies to frozen food.

Salad and other vegetables stay fresher and retain their nutritional value better when stored in a cool, dark, well-ventilated place. Refrigerators prolong their shelf life but they should be well wrapped to prevent wilting. Buy vegetables and fruit when they are in season. Fresh fruit and vegetables are usually the cheapest but in late spring frozen vegetables may be useful.

Store food carefully to prevent deterioration. Ensure that the fridge is operating below 5°C. It may be useful to buy a fridge thermometer to check. Put food away quickly in the fridge. Opening the door warms up the interior temperature as does putting warm food straight into the fridge. Defrosting the fridge and freezer regularly will help to keep them running efficiently and effectively.

Reading Food Labels

By law, a food label has to provide information about the product: what it is (for example 'baked beans in tomato sauce'), its country of origin, the name and address of the manufacturer or distributor and the net weight or volume of the contents. It must also provide information about its safe usage: how it should be stored, how it should be cooked or reconstituted and how soon it should be eaten. The time before which the food should be eaten will be indicated as a 'use by date' or a 'best before date'.

A use by date is found on perishable fresh foods such as meat, poultry, fish and some dairy products. Items should be used by this date to minimize the risk of food poisoning. Once the use by date has been passed, it should be assumed that the food is not safe to eat. It is an offence to sell foods after their use by date.

A best before date is found on foods with a longer shelf life (such as breakfast cereals, canned goods and frozen goods). After this date, some texture or flavour quality may be lost but the product will still be safe to eat. The exception to this is eggs, which carry a best before date, but actually have to be sold one week before this date. Eggs should not be used after their best before date.

Finally, the label must also carry a list of the ingredients used to make the product. These are given in descending order of content. If water is given as the first ingredient then water is there in the largest amount. However, the list may not give the actual amounts of each ingredient. It is possible that the first ingredient may make up the bulk of the product and all other ingredients are only present in very small amounts.

Nutritional labelling is not compulsory although most manufacturers and retailers do provide it voluntarily on the vast majority of products. If nutrition information is given, it has to be given in an order that is laid down by legislation:

- Energy in kilojoules (kJ) or kilocalories (kcal)
- Protein in grams (g)
- Carbohydrate in grams (g)
- Fat in grams (g)

More detailed nutritional information can be given in the following format:

- Energy (kJ/kcal)
- Protein (g)
- Carbohydrate (g)
  of which sugars (g)

- Fat (g)
  of which saturates (g)
- Fibre (g)
- Sodium (g)

The rules for labelling vitamins and minerals are more complex. These can only be given if the food provides a significant proportion of the Recommended Daily Amount (RDA) for each vitamin and mineral as defined by European legislation.

Legislation requires nutritional information to be given per 100g or per 100ml of product, although consumers will usually prefer the information to be per serving, and manufacturers often provide this extra information. Until recently the information on labels has not really helped consumers to know what they are actually eating. The Department of Health has now produced daily guideline intakes for the average adult. These can only be approximate figures but they do give some indication of the target figures for the general public, although they will not always be appropriate for athletes.

Daily Guideline Intakes		
	Men	*Women*
Energy (as calories)	2,500kcal	2,000kcal
Fat	95g	70g
Saturates	30g	20g
Sugar	70g	50g
Fibre	20g	16g
Sodium	2.5g	2g

Nutrition Claims

Although there are some legal constraints on the nutritional claims that manufacturers can make (such as reduced fat or low sugar) this area is still not well regulated. Many manufacturers follow a voluntary code of practice.

If a nutritional claim is made the label must provide nutritional labelling information.

'Reduced in' and 'low in' are not the same. For example, foods 'low in' fat will contain less than foods 'reduced in' fat. 'Reduced' or 'low' does not mean 'none'. Only foods labelled as, for example, 'fat free' will contain minimal amounts of fat. Foods flagged as being 'rich in' will contain more of a particular nutrient than foods declaring they are 'a source of'.

Cooking

Overcooking food can destroy nutrients, particularly vitamins as most are sensitive to heat, light, water or air. However losses can be minimized by correct storage and cooking. Excessive cooking can also reduce the appeal of food as colour, flavour and texture can be lost – meat becomes tough, sauces dry out and rice and pasta stick together.

Vegetables should be prepared just before cooking. Soaking them in water should be avoided, particularly after chopping, as vitamins will leach out into the water. Vegetables should be prepared in large rather than small pieces to help minimize vitamin losses. Wherever possible skins should not be removed as these provide fibre and vitamins are often concentrated just under the skin.

Vegetables should be cooked in the shortest possible time and in the minimum amount of water. Apart from retaining valuable nutrients, it keeps the colour bright and texture crunchy. Microwaving, stir-frying or steaming vegetables are all excellent ways of helping to retain nutrients. Cooked vegetables should be eaten as soon as possible after cooking.

Fresh vegetables and fruit should be bought regularly as vitamins will be lost on storage. Frozen vegetables often have a higher vitamin content than fresh but this can be lost if they are not cooked properly. Frozen vegetables should be cooked from frozen, not allowed to thaw out, and added directly to boiling water. Check the storage dates of frozen vegetables to make sure they are not out of date.

Raw fruit and vegetables should be eaten whenever possible for maximum nutritional benefit.

Speeding Things Up
Some athletes enjoy spending time in the kitchen, finding it relaxing and a profitable way of unwinding. For others it is a chore and only viewed as a means to an end, refuelling. For those who want to minimize kitchen time but also want to improve their diet, the following may be useful tips.

- Canned chopped tomatoes rather than canned whole ones take less time to break down when cooking sauces.
- Using cooked ham instead of bacon in sauces or fillings for jacket potatoes cuts down cooking time and the number of cooking pans used.
- Small mushrooms can be added whole to sauces, saving preparation time.
- Grate a large amount of cheese then freeze it in 'topping-sized' amounts. It won't need thawing out if used to melt on top of pizzas or to be stirred into sauces.
- Breadcrumbs freeze well and can be used straight from the freezer for topping and coating food.
- Packets of savoury rice make a good base for risottos to which cooked meat and fresh or frozen vegetables can be added.
- Baking potatoes in their skins (unless using a microwave) can be speeded up by baking two smaller ones rather than one large one. A skewer through the potato helps to transmit heat to the centre so that it cooks faster.
- Frozen fruit juice defrosts more quickly if blended first in a food processor.

- Cook double the amount of pasta or rice required to provide the basis of a cold salad for the next day. It should be stored in the fridge but kept no longer than one day.
- Microwave cooking is considerably quicker than other cooking methods. Nutritionally it is a good way to cook. More vitamins are retained when cooking in a microwave oven than virtually any other cooking method and because it is a moist method of cooking, addition of fat is not normally needed to prevent sticking. It also saves on washing up and cleaning.

Relieving the Boredom

It is all too easy to keep cooking the same foods and then to find that boredom has set in. Similar foods can be livened up by just adding an extra ingredient, such as a different herb added to a pasta sauce or a mixture of spices instead of the standard curry powder. The label on a jar of herbs or spices will often make suggestions.

Dijon mustard stirred into yoghurt warmed over a low heat makes an interesting sauce to which vegetables, ham or chicken pieces can be added before pouring over a plate of pasta.

Vary the shape and colour of the pasta used, and alternate between fresh and dried varieties. Try out new varieties of bread and breakfast cereals to avoid monotony.

Food Safety

Improper handling and storage of food and leftovers is one of the most common causes of food poisoning in the home and a bout of diarrhoea and vomiting will play havoc with training schedules or, worse still, competition. Too often the papers tell of a sportsperson who has been unable to play or compete because of food poisoning.

Raw meat and poultry must not come into contact with cooked or ready to eat foods. Drips from raw food must not fall onto other foods, including foods in the salad drawer. Uncooked foods should be on the lowest shelves of the fridge. Cooked and uncooked foods should never be on the same shelves.

When handling foods, it is important that hands are clean and that they are washed between handling raw foods and cooked or ready to eat foods. Knives and other kitchen utensils should also be washed between handling raw and cooked foods.

Hands should always be washed after going to the toilet and after handling pets. Domestic pets should be kept out of the kitchen if possible but certainly away from food, dishes and worktops. Working surfaces should be washed thoroughly and often. Chopping boards need special attention as they can lead to the transfer of infection from one kind of food to another. Cooked or ready to eat foods should not be placed on a surface that has just had raw foods on it.

Thawing and cooking instructions on frozen foods should be read and followed carefully. It is particularly important that meat and poultry are completely thawed before cooking. After thawing frozen raw poultry, there should be no ice particles and the flesh should be soft and pliable. Foods should not be re-frozen once thawed unless they have been thoroughly cooked.

Food should be cooked well, instructions on packs should be followed and when food is reheated it should be heated until piping hot. Leftovers should be cooled quickly in a shallow dish, covered and then put into the fridge or freezer immediately (within two hours). Putting hot food straight into the fridge will cause the temperature to rise and encourage condensation and possible contamination of other foods. As a general rule, leftovers kept in the fridge should be eaten within two days.

Hot foods should be kept hot and cold

foods cold. Sounds simple but it is all too easy to leave food standing around. Cooked food should only be reheated once whether cooked in the kitchen or bought as a cook chill product. Any food left over after reheating must be thrown away.

Vegetables, salads and fruits should be washed in clean cold running water.

It is not advisable to eat food containing uncooked eggs.

If using dried beans, including dried red kidney beans, it is important to soak the beans in water for up to twelve hours (or overnight), throw away the water and then boil them briskly in fresh water for at least ten minutes. This destroys the toxin in the raw beans. Canned beans which have already been properly cooked in processing can be used straight from the can.

If canned food is used and there is some left over, it should be emptied into a bowl or plastic container, covered and stored in the fridge, not kept in the can. Leftovers of questionable age and safety should never be tasted. If a leftover has been stored for too long or if it looks or smells peculiar, it should be thrown away.

Meal Timing

Regardless of the amount of food that is required, athletes should spread their food intake throughout the day as four, five or even six eating occasions. The actual timing of each eating occasion will be determined by individual factors such as work, college or school timetables, timing of training sessions, nutritional requirements, travelling time from the various destinations and personal preferences and eating habits.

Eating before training must be timed so as to leave the athlete feeling comfortable once the training session starts with no stomach discomfort, nausea or bloatedness. Refuelling after training must take place as soon as possible after training finishes. This may be a refuelling drink and snack or it may be a meal.

Athletes with particularly high energy demands will usually need a pre-bedtime light meal, often resembling another breakfast. The advice in this book should enable athletes to build up their own diet plans to meet both nutritional and practical individual requirements. In most cases individual diet plans will probably include a breakfast, midday meal and evening meal with one or two refuelling snacks (based on the carbohydrate requirement post-training) and possibly a further light meal in the late evening.

Breakfast for All

Breakfast tends to be a matter of habit, but habits are not always good ones. Many athletes have high energy requirements and habitually missing meals means that those extra nutritional demands are unlikely to be met. Breakfast is a meal which is often skipped.

While asleep, the average person moves sixty to seventy times a night with a dozen full turns. This uses up energy at an average rate of 80kcal per hour. As food is not taken on board during the night, this energy requirement is met by using the body's stores. By morning, blood sugar and insulin levels, which can influence mood and mental performance, are often low and energy stores need to be replaced. If breakfast is missed, a substantial mid-morning high carbohydrate light meal of sandwiches, rolls, cereal bars, bananas and so on will be needed. Various suggestions for breakfast ideas are given in Appendix 2.

Training and Breakfast

For athletes who train early in the morning, timing breakfast may be a problem. Some athletes can eat breakfast and train soon after without any ill effects, although this may depend on the type and intensity of the training. Others manage a small breakfast and have the bulk of the meal straight after training. The typical breakfast of cereal and toast is ideal for refuelling as it is low in fat and high in carbohydrate.

There are some athletes who can train without breakfast and still put in a good session but others will feel weak and light-headed if training before eating. However, training is all about teaching the body to do things it has not been able to do before, such as lift heavier weights, run faster or for longer. It is also possible to teach the body to get used to having breakfast and then training soon after. Going from no food at all to eating a large bowl of cereal and a pile of toast before training is likely to lead to disaster but starting with small amounts and building up the intake gradually will not.

The following plan is suggested: on waking, use the bathroom, then eat half a slice of toast and a small glass of fruit juice. Then change into training kit and warm up and stretch before starting the training session. This gives the maximum time between eating breakfast and starting training so that any discomfort should be negligible. With time the amount eaten can be increased. Early morning training sessions should become better for having eaten breakfast.

Midday Meals

Midday meals may take the form of a packed meal prepared at home and taken to work, college, school or the training venue or bought in a local sandwich bar. Packed lunch ideas are given in Appendix 2. Lunch may be a cooked meal prepared at home in which case it can be tailor-made to nutritional demands and personal preferences. The main problems will be for those athletes who have to rely on canteen food or whose work involves a fair amount of lunchtime entertaining. Fortunately, many workplace canteens are moving towards providing lower fat options. Practical advice about eating out can be found in Chapter 13.

Evening Meals

Again, the majority of evening meals will probably be eaten at home, either prepared for the athlete by a partner or family member or by the athlete him or herself on return from work or training. If training has been late, coming home and having to start preparing a meal is tough for the exhausted athlete. However it is important to remember that it is better to eat late at night than not at all as the refuelling process is vital. This is particularly so when there is a morning training session to look forward to.

Not every evening meal has to be based on pasta, rice, potatoes, with meat, fish or poultry and two cooked vegetables but it does have to provide plenty of carbohydrate, some protein and not much fat. The following are some quick high carbohydrate meals that can be prepared in minutes and will be infinitely better than a stop-over at the local fast food outlet.

- A large can of spaghetti in tomato sauce on toast or pitta bread.
- A large can of baked beans in tomato sauce on toast.
- Warmed pitta bread piled with baked beans, topped with grated cheese and grilled to melt the cheese.
- A pile of honey and banana sandwiches.
- Pitta bread spread with low fat soft cheese and filled with canned, drained sweetcorn and red kidney beans.
- Lentil, thick vegetable or minestrone soup with lots of bread or toast.
- Toasted muffins with low fat soft cheese and bananas.
- Pitta bread with hummus.
- For microwave users: jacket potatoes

(several small potatoes rather than one big one) with tuna and sweetcorn or baked beans.

- A quick pizza made with a large thick pizza base, traditional Ragu or Dolmio sauce, a can of sweetcorn and some grated cheese. Pizza bases can be defrosted under the grill or in a microwave. Spread the warmed base with the tomato sauce, sprinkle sweetcorn on top, followed by the grated cheese and warm under the grill until the cheese is bubbling.
- Cooked pasta with sauce. Fresh pasta is more expensive than dried but quicker to cook. The sauce may be a tomato-based sauce (such as Ragu) warmed through with drained, canned beans, sweetcorn or peas. Alternatively, use a sauce of melted low fat soft cheese (such as Philadelphia Light or Shape) with assorted cooked vegetables and a few chopped nuts. Another option is a sauce of chopped onions, canned tomatoes, garlic and herbs, topped with a little Parmesan cheese.

If all else fails, a large bowl of breakfast cereal with chopped banana, sugar (if desired) and semi-skimmed milk will certainly go some way to refuelling.

Further ideas for more elaborate meals can be found in Appendix 2 – but no recipes. There is no shortage of recipe books that promise meals in ten, twenty or thirty minutes. Using the advice in this book, athletes should be able to pick out the most suitable recipes and with time learn to adapt less suitable ones so they really can eat well and perform better.

CHAPTER 5
The Competition Diet

The consequences of starting competition dehydrated and with inadequate glycogen stores will be a poor performance and a disappointing result. General advice in the days prior to competition are to taper training, incorporate a rest day, consume a high carbohydrate diet (but not to exceed the energy requirement for the reduced level of exercise) and maintain a regular fluid intake. Such advice may suit a marathon runner but it is not appropriate for a footballer with one or even two matches interspersed in each week's training schedule.

Many of the principles of the competition diet are the same as those for training and will therefore apply to all athletes, but the practical advice will vary according to the sport and competition conditions.

CARBOHYDRATE LOADING

Continuous moderate to high intensity exercise for more than 90 minutes results in glycogen depletion, when athletes feel exhausted and can no longer keep up their pace. This happens around the 20-mile mark in the marathon and is commonly called

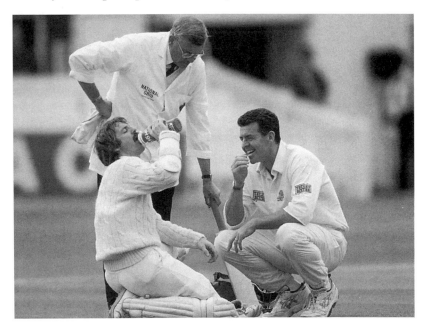

England's Jack Russell (left) takes a drink from physiotherapist Wayne Morton as umpire Dickie Bird inspects his bat.

'hitting the wall'. The cycling equivalent is known as 'bonking'. Carbohydrate loading is by no means a new technique. The original research firmly establishing the relationship between a high carbohydrate diet and improved endurance capacity was reported in 1939. Subsequent studies clearly showed that the amount of stored glycogen increased to higher than normal values when a high carbohydrate diet was eaten during recovery from exhaustive exercise or after glycogen stores had been depleted.

Traditional carbohydrate loading is achieved by first exercising to exhaustion to reduce the muscle glycogen level. This is then followed by three days on a low carbohydrate diet (high in protein and fat). For the last three days before the race, a high carbohydrate diet providing at least 70 per cent of total energy as carbohydrate is consumed. Carbohydrate loading does not increase initial speed during endurance events but it does delay the onset of fatigue. Improved race times can be attributed to this delay, allowing athletes to maintain a higher intensity of exertion for a longer period of time.

The wisdom of exercising to exhaustion followed by eating a low carbohydrate diet has been questioned in recent years. Exercising to exhaustion so close to competition can cause premature peaking, interfere with the training programme and increase the risk of injury. The low carbohydrate diet is unpleasant and causes irritability and light-headedness, making training very difficult. All these factors can seriously undermine confidence at a time when the athlete is preparing for competition. On returning to a high carbohydrate diet, athletes often experience digestive problems. It is also easy to get the loading wrong by not eating enough carbohydrate to supersaturate the muscles with glycogen, so all that effort and unpleasantness is to no avail.

Many athletes now adopt a modified loading technique. Training is progressively tapered in the week leading up to the race with complete rest the day before the race. At the same time, the carbohydrate content of the diet is increased to provide at least 70 per cent of the total energy. In practical terms, this means aiming for 8 to 10g carbohydrate per kg body weight. For many athletes this will just mean a slight increase on an already high carbohydrate training diet. It is important not to increase the overall intake of calories, as training is tapered. Simply cutting back fat intake and making protein food portions slightly smaller will achieve this. Following a modified loading technique can double muscle glycogen levels without any of the drawbacks of the traditional method.

Because water is stored with glycogen (three parts water to one part glycogen) some weight gain is experienced. The extra stored water may be helpful in compensating for fluid losses through sweating, although it may cause stiffness, muscle cramps and heaviness in the legs initially. Carbohydrate loading is

---

Who Might Benefit From Loading?

Yes	No
Marathon runners	Track and field athletes
Long distance swimmers	Swimmers
Cross country skiers	Downhill skiers
Triathletes	Rowers
Long distance cyclists	Footballers
	Rugby players
	Weight lifters

Caution: Carbohydrate loading may not be appropriate for diabetic athletes and those with raised blood triglycerides. Such athletes should seek medical advice.

of no value for events lasting less than 90 minutes.

Pre-Competition

Planning the competition diet should begin, in most cases, the day before competition and particularly with the last meal of the day before. For competitions taking place early in the day, this will be the last opportunity to really top up the muscle glycogen stores. The meal should contain only familiar foods, with emphasis on carbohydrate-rich foods but a de-emphasis on fibre-rich sources of carbohydrates. Pre-competition nerves and tension will be a more efficient bowel mover. Athletes who have problems eating on competition days must take extra care over this meal. Fluid intakes should be maintained at a high level, particularly if the competition day is forecast to be warm and/or humid.

Pre-Event

The pre-event meal has several functions:

- To top up the fuel stores of liver glycogen after the fast of the night.
- To top up stores of muscle glycogen
- To prevent hunger pangs and leave the stomach feeling settled and comfortable.
- To maintain hydration in the run up to the competition.
- To give the athlete peace of mind. Knowing that the planned dietary and fluid preparation have been completed can help psychologically.

The meal should be made up of low fat, low or moderate protein and low fibre/high carbohydrate foods. This will ensure that the food has left the stomach (fat and protein take longer to leave the stomach than carbohydrate) and been digested before the start of competition. A large meal normally takes three to four hours to digest, a smaller meal two to three hours and a snack one to two hours, but nerves can often cause a delay in digestion. Liquid meals such as Build Up can help because they empty from the stomach more quickly than solid food and any nausea is usually reduced.

Athletes competing in sports involving running or physical contact will probably need to allow more digestion time, or certainly stomach emptying time, than athletes whose body weight is supported while they are competing.

It is important that athletes select foods they like and feel comfortable eating and that the time of the meal also suits them. This can be discovered by trial and error during training and minor competitions. A new regime should never be tried for the first time on a major competition day. Carbohydrate intakes to aim for are 1 to 4g per kg body weight one to four hours prior to the start of competition. This

---

Suitable Pre-Competition Items

Baked beans or spaghetti in tomato sauce on toast.
Low fibre breakfast cereal with low fat milk.
Banana, jam, honey or marmalade sandwiches or on toast.
Crumpets, pancakes, muffins with honey, jam or marmalade.
Bagels, baguettes or sandwiches with lean cold meat, tuna or salmon.
Jacket potatoes with low fat toppings such as baked beans, cottage or low fat soft cheese, tuna and sweetcorn.
Low fat milk shakes or smoothies.
Cereal bars, breakfast bars (Nutrigrains) or Squares.
Mullerice and Mullerlight yoghurt.
Bananas.
Isotonic sports drinks.

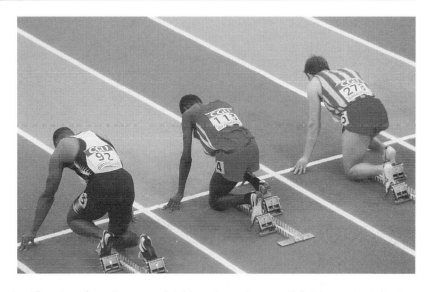

(left to right) Mensah Elliott, Luke Gittens and Nigel Taylor on the start line for a heat of the men's 60m hurdles.

means, for example, 4g if eating four hours before the competition, 1g if there is only one hour before the competition starts.

MARATHON RUNNING

Within the scope of this book it is impossible to give precise practical advice to cover all competitive sporting situations. Marathon running is probably not a competitive sport for the vast majority of those who take part (just an incentive to keep fit, raise money or get out into the open air with like-minded people) but dietary preparation is none the less vital in preventing injury, heat stress and perhaps helping to make the day more enjoyable. The following advice will therefore be of use to all marathon runners and can be adapted to suit other sports and competitions.

Countdown to Marathon Day

In the last two or three months before the marathon the longest runs should be used to practise the fluid count-down procedure. It is only by doing this that runners will get used to drinking the volumes of fluid required during the race to minimize dehydration and gain confidence to follow the same strategy on the day. It is also vital that runners have a dress rehearsal for the day itself. Those who have done all their training runs later in the day may find getting up at crack of dawn, having breakfast when they would normally still be asleep and then running early in the morning (when most marathons start) a shock to their system. Going through the routine beforehand could knock minutes off the finishing time on the day.

The Final Four Days Before Competition

As training tapers down, the proportion of carbohydrate in the diet should be increased without increasing the overall amount of food (calories) eaten. Three meals a day will be needed, interspersed with snacks at mid-morning, mid-afternoon and near bedtime. Breakfast provides a great opportunity to eat the right foods, such as cereals, bread and preserves, together with plenty of fluids including fruit juice and milk. Lunch can be built around starchy carbohydrates such as banana or low fat soft cheese sandwiches, jacket potatoes with tuna, cottage cheese or baked beans, pasta and rice salads or a simple pasta and tomato dish, finishing with fruit and yoghurt and more fluids. The evening meal can be more of the same but adding a small amount of lean meat, chicken or fish and maybe starting with a thick vegetable soup with bread and finishing with fruit crumble and custard or a milk pudding. This may seem like a lot of food but portions will vary considerably between runners.

Running a marathon does use up a large amount of energy. At this stage it is important to have foods that are familiar. For runners staying at home or with friends this will not be a problem but for those who have to travel and stay in hotels or bed and breakfast accommodation care will be needed. Familiar food eaten in hygienic places is an important component of successful marathon preparation.

Sufficient fluids should be drunk to ensure that runners are fully hydrated by the day of the race. Urine ought to be pale in colour and plentiful, especially in the evenings. A pee chart can be a particularly useful monitoring tool in the days leading up to the race. A change of routine when away from home can lead to a reduction in the amount of fluid being drunk.

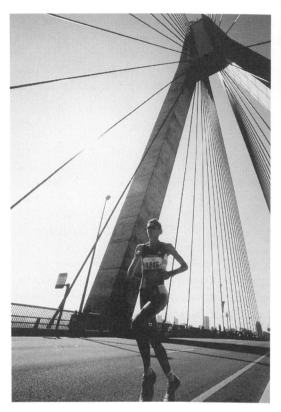

Great Britain's Marian Sutton crosses the Anzak bridge in the Sydney 2000 Olympic Marathon.

The Day Before the Race

Breakfast and lunch can be similar to the previous days but if any meals are eaten out, care must be taken to avoid unfamiliar, under-cooked and potentially risky items such as spicy foods, seafood, fatty food, rare meat and gas-producers such as beans. Meat should not be high on the menu and certainly not hot-dogs, hamburgers and kebabs. Upset tummies cause dehydration which could develop into a serious health problem during the marathon. This should be a restful day so many runners will not need snacks. There is no need to overeat at the evening meal, and indeed appetite may be reduced due to excitement or nerves. Portions should be normal with the emphasis, of course, on carbohydrates, so good choices would be pasta with tomato sauce or a tomato and vegetable topped pizza with very little cheese. Extra bread, fruit or yoghurt to finish and lots of fluids will help to maximize the muscle glycogen stores.

Fluid intake should be kept up until just before bed. Alcohol is a diuretic and in most situations the recommendation would be to avoid alcohol at this stage. In practice, some runners find that a small drink is relaxing (particularly when sleeping in unfamiliar surroundings). In this case having no more than one pint (half for females) of ordinary beer or lager (no strong varieties) will not be a problem but spirits and wine should be avoided. Having a long non-alcoholic drink afterwards will counter any dehydrating effects of the alcohol.

The Morning of the Race

Breakfast should be planned well in advance. Runners staying away from home must find what foods will be available early in the morning (perhaps as early as 5.30am). Not all accommodation will be able to provide a meal at this time, especially if the race takes place on a Sunday. If there is any doubt about what will be available, runners should take their own emergency supplies, including any dishes or utensils that might be needed. Fortunately suitable foods travel well and do not present any major storage or preparation problems. Plenty of fluids should be drunk with breakfast and intake kept up by taking frequent sips of water or a sports drink (whichever has been found best during training) all the way to the starting area.

Thirty to Forty-Five Minutes Before the Start

A visit to the loo approximately thirty to forty-five minutes before the start of the marathon should be made to both urinate and defecate. This is important as both factors may influence drinking behaviour during the race. It may be necessary to think ahead and start queuing early to get the timing right. The warm-up and stretching session then follows.

Five Minutes Before the Start

Drinking 300 to 600ml of fluid (water or a sports drink) can help to prevent dehydration but this is a technique that must have been practised during training runs. There is no time for the urine to form before the race starts and once running, blood flow to the kidneys is reduced so that urine formation becomes minimal. It takes confidence to do this on race

day and thus experimenting in training is vital. Some runners eat a high carbohydrate snack at this stage but this should also be tried in training beforehand. Suitable snacks include Turkish delight, mint cake or other pure sugary sources of carbohydrate.

During the Race

Fluids should be drunk at every available opportunity, ideally aiming for about 150ml every fifteen minutes. Runners can measure this out at home to see what this volume looks like. Fluids must be drunk early on in the race to counter the fluid losses that will occur in the later stages of the race. Runners who wait until they feel thirsty and start to dehydrate before they drink simply won't be able to absorb enough fluids. The race will be over before the fluids start to do any good. Runners must not be tempted to drink anything during the race that has not been tried and tested in training. The race itself is not the time to experiment with a new sports drink.

After the Race

Refuelling and rehydrating must start as soon as possible after runners cross the line. Many runners will want to celebrate with alcohol but this should be delayed at least until full rehydration has been achieved.

MULTI-EVENT COMPETITIONS

Athletes who are competing several times on the same day need to keep up their carbohydrate intake to maintain the glycogen stores. This needs a strategy, with specific foods and fluids taken at specific times. What and when will depend on the length of the event, intensity of the exercise and the length of time before the next event.

Timing of Pre-Event Meals

Early Morning Event (8.00am)
High carbohydrate meal with plenty of fluids the night before.
Light snack about two hours before (high carbohydrate, familiar foods).
Fluids from then on.

Mid-Morning Event (10.00am)
High carbohydrate meal with plenty of fluids the night before.
Normal breakfast three hours before.
Fluids from then on.

Mid-Afternoon Event (3.00pm)
High carbohydrate meal with plenty of fluids the night before.
Normal breakfast on getting up.
Light snack two to three hours before (high carbohydrate, familiar foods).
Fluids from then on.

Evening Event (7.30pm)
High carbohydrate breakfast with plenty of fluids.
High carbohydrate lunch with fluids.
Light snack two to three hours before (high carbohydrate, familiar foods).
Fluids from then on.

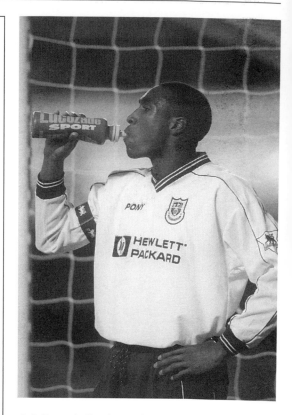

Sol Campbell takes a drink.

Sports drinks can help boost the carbohydrate intake at any time around competition.

If there is one hour or less between events, consume carbohydrate in liquid form (sports drinks, juices) or easily digested solid food (bananas and other fresh, canned and dried fruits) to ensure no cramps or gut distress. The amount should be limited to what feels comfortable.

If there are two or three hours between events, eat items such as plain bagels, pancakes, cereal with or without milk, fruit or sports drinks. Items that are enjoyed pre-competition are also likely to be suitable for this time.

If there are four or more hours between events, eat enjoyable meals with a strong emphasis on the carbohydrate content.

TEAM SPORTS

Taking on board fluids during competition is permitted within the rules and regulations of many sports, particularly racquet sports. The opportunities to drink during team sports such as football, rugby, hockey, netball and cricket are much fewer and dictated by the rules of each individual sport. Players must be encouraged to use every opportunity to drink that presents during the match, such as official breaks (quarters and half time) and stoppages (injuries, substitutions, changes of batsmen or goal kicks). Teams should work out strategies to get fluids onto the pitch quickly at every opportunity and to target players who are known to dehydrate easily.

POST-COMPETITION

Refuelling and rehydrating is as important after competition as after training and the same practical advice applies. Athletes taking part in competitions or tournaments which continue over several days must be meticulous about restocking their glycogen stores and restoring full hydration status at the end of each day. If the competition venue is away from home, athletes should take a supply of suitable snacks and drinks in case the food provided at the venue or accommodation falls short of requirements.

CHAPTER 6

Weight Loss, Weight Gain and Making Weight

Some athletes inherit physical characteristics making them potential naturals for a sport. Height is obviously an advantage in sports such as volleyball and basketball. Arm reach is an asset in boxing. Body weight is an important factor in rugby when it comes to scrummaging because it is difficult for forwards to shove back a heavier opposing pack. However it is still better to have this weight as muscle rather than fat.

In a few sports, particularly skill sports such as archery, darts, snooker and golf, body weight and composition do not appear to matter. However, overweight athletes competing in hot or humid climates may feel uncomfortable and as a consequence not produce their best performance.

LOSING WEIGHT

Athletes wish to reduce body weight for several reasons: to improve performance, to enhance their appearance or to compete at a particular weight (known as 'making weight'). Before embarking on a weight reduction programme, the following should be considered:

- Is a reduction in body weight/body fat necessary?
- Will a reduction improve performance?
- What is a realistic weight or body composition for the individual athlete?
- What is the best way to achieve the desired/agreed goals?

Losing too much weight or losing it too quickly can have a negative effect on performance. A gradual reduction in body weight/body fat through diet and training will allow the athlete together with the coach, fitness expert and sports dietitian or nutritionist to monitor the effect the loss is having on performance. In this way excessive weight loss or too rapid weight loss can be avoided and risk of any loss in performance minimized. Making weight is a very different scenario and will be addressed later.

The Truth About Weight Loss

The science behind weight loss is not complicated and can be summed up by these simple equations:

Energy intake = Energy output → Weight is maintained

Energy intake > Energy output → Weight is gained

Energy intake < Energy output → Weight is lost

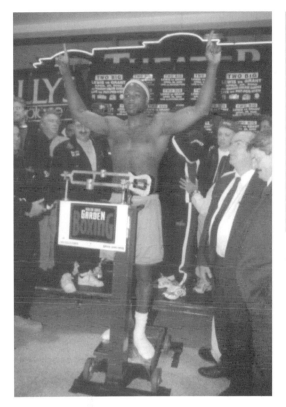

Lennox Lewis at the weigh-in.

If the energy intake from food and drink does not meet total energy requirements the body has to draw on its own energy stores. If the energy intake is reduced slowly without too severe a restriction, body fat will be used to make up the energy shortfall. If energy intake is cut back drastically, glycogen and muscle protein will also be used. This could limit training, resulting in reduction in energy output and an increased risk of injury.

Dieting Myths

Many of the currently trendy diets are based on a high protein, low carbohydrate intake (examples are The Zone diet and Dr Atkin's New Diet Revolution). These diets can reduce weight in the short-term (because energy intake is reduced) but they obviously cannot support a training or exercise programme for any period of time.

'Food combining' has been popular for decades. It is based on the rationale that carbohydrate and protein should not be eaten at the same meal. This ignores the fact that the digestive system is capable of digesting foods containing both nutrients at the same time (*see* Chapter 2) and that a wide selection of foods contain both carbohydrate and protein. Successful weight loss by this method is only due to the limit on food intake imposed by the restrictions of the diet and therefore the reduction in the overall energy intake. Again, the carbohydrate intake of this diet will not be sufficient to meet the requirements of a training programme.

What About Fat-Burning Exercise?

Fat makes its greatest contribution as an energy source in low to moderate intensity exercise. Many people therefore believe they must exercise at a low intensity to increase fat burning and lose weight. In fact, high intensity exercise is probably more helpful to less intense exercise as a means of controlling body weight. As exercise intensity increases, the energy cost becomes greater, resulting a bigger energy deficit. Those who exercise at a low intensity invariably fail to exercise long enough to reach a similar energy deficit. It is not the proportion of fat used as a fuel but the rate of fuel utilization which is the key to loss of body fat through exercise. The optimum fat-burning intensity is therefore the intensity at which an individual can comfortably expend the greatest amount of energy, bearing in mind the time available to exercise.

The Weight Loss Plan

Sensible, achievable targets for body fat and body weight must be set and this may require the help of a sports dietitian or exercise physiologist. A reduction in energy intake of 500 to 1,000kcal per day will produce a steady weight loss while still ensuring an adequate energy and nutrient intake to support training and maintain health and general well being. A daily energy intake of less than 1,200 to 1,500kcal should not be followed without the help and advice of a sports dietitian.

The simplest way to achieve the energy deficit is to reduce the intake of calorie-dense items, particularly fat and alcohol, while maintaining the intake of protein and carbohydrate. High fibre foods will supply carbohydrate but will also help to keep hunger at bay because of their bulking properties. Much of the advice in Chapter 4 together with the following suggestions should help athletes to draw up their weight loss plans.

Keeping a food diary for a week can highlight inappropriate food choices, poor eating patterns and boredom eating. Noting what, when and how much was eaten and where, who with and while doing what, it should be possible to identify problem and danger areas. For example, unhealthy snacks may be eaten while relaxing in front of the television.

Females may be eating similar portions to their male partners, even though their energy requirements are less. Boredom, habit or mood may affect intake.

Eating irregularly is not the way to lose weight. There should be no long gaps between eating. Those who skip meals are more likely to overeat later in the day. The classic excuse of not having eaten all day can result in an excessive intake of energy in a short space of time in the evening. This is rather like filling the car up with petrol and then putting it in the garage, instead of filling up before a journey. Eating regularly through the day provides the body with fuel when it needs it and will use it rather than storing it up.

Breakfast should not be missed as it boosts the blood glucose and energy levels and helps to prevent snacking on inappropriate foods during the morning.

Fruit and vegetables are important as they are packed with essential vitamins and minerals but low in calories. Eating more fruit and drinking less fruit juice can help to keep the calories down without compromising the intake of essential nutrients and phytochemicals.

Fluid intake remains very important and low calorie squashes and water (tap, mineral or flavoured) will help to keep calorie intake down. Those athletes who use sports drinks should continue to use them in the period before, during and immediately after exercising but not at other times. Drinking water or low calorie drinks before and during meals can help make meals more filling.

Small amounts of favourite foods as a treat now and again can help to keep the dieting momentum going without abandoning the diet completely.

Athletes who tend to increase weight during the off-season and then struggle to lose it again at the start of pre-season training should find some of the advice in this chapter helpful. There is no suggestion that a strict diet should be followed at this time, only that keeping some control over intake while output is reduced will make pre-season training a little easier.

GAINING WEIGHT

When athletes express a desire to gain weight it is actually muscle mass that they wish to increase. This requires a well-designed resistance training programme, an energy intake that will leave the athlete in positive balance (energy in > energy out) and adequate rest and recovery time. For some athletes this seems like an impossible struggle and, in some cases, it may be. Looking at the physical build of other family members may give an indication of what can be expected. Again, much of the advice in Chapter 4 together with the following suggestions should help athletes to draw up their own weight gain plans.

Following a progressive resistance training programme will help to stimulate muscle growth. Aiming to increase daily energy intake by 500kcal per day, more in some cases, should produce a steady, but invariably slow weight increase. The extra energy must be sufficient to cover the cost of building new tissue and the extra energy cost of the resistance training programme. Regular meal patterns with snacks interspersed in between can be built up to six or more meal occasions. Meals should never be skipped, including breakfast.

Although weight increase is the goal, this is not an excuse to eat high fat foods. The emphasis must still be on plenty of carbohydrate for energy and protein, vitamins and minerals for the growth and support of new tissue. Intake of bulky foods should be minimized, concentrating instead on high-energy nutrient-dense foods. Portion sizes should be big but must not cause any internal distress.

Drinking high energy drinks (fruit juices, milk, milkshakes or smoothies) rather than tea or coffee can push energy intake up but it is better to drink them between rather than with meals. They can be quite filling and if drunk with meals could result in less food being eaten and thus no significant increase in the overall energy intake.

If weight gain is very slow or non-existent it is worth keeping a food diary. Too often athletes believe they are eating well but a carefully kept food diary shows otherwise. Often those who seem unable to gain weight are also the very people who are not enormously interested in food. They may miss meals without being aware of it. Keeping a food diary can be a revelation.

Supplements for Weight Gain

A variety of supplements promoted to increase muscle mass are marketed to athletes. These include chromium, creatine, vanadyl sulphate, boron, beta-hydroxy-beta-methyl-butyrate (HMB), protein powders and amino acids. However, chromium, vanadium and boron have not been found to increase muscle mass and sufficient protein can be derived from the diet without the use of protein supplements and amino acids.

HMB is a metabolite of the amino acid leucine and is also found in some foods including citrus fruit. Not an essential nutrient, the function of HMB in the body is not fully understood. It has been suggested that HMB increases muscle mass by preventing the breakdown of muscle protein after intense resistance training and by enhancing the repair process. The few studies that have been undertaken support this theory. More studies are needed, particularly to determine long-term safety. Nevertheless it is a popular supplement amongst many athletes.

Creatine (which will be covered in more detail in Chapter 7) is another amino acid which occurs naturally in the diet and which has been shown to increase body weight. Short-term increases appear to be due to water retention rather than an increase in muscle mass. However creatine allows a greater amount of high intensity work to be undertaken in training, resulting in a greater training response which, long-term, would be expected to increase muscle mass.

MAKING WEIGHT

Most athletes know that they perform best at a particular weight or at least within a narrow range of weights. In some sports, athletes have to compete at a particular weight, which is often considerably lighter than their natural weight. To achieve these goals they may follow strict diets or rely on various rapid weight loss techniques. This is known as 'making weight' – the athlete must weigh a certain amount in order to make a weight class prior to competition. Sports where this practice takes place include boxing, martial arts, weight lifting, wrestling and lightweight rowing and horse racing.

In most sports, weight classes are intended to eliminate injuries which might arise if competitors are ill matched physically or to allow athletes of all sizes to compete on an equal basis. Unfortunately, some athletes lose weight to qualify for a lower weight class in the belief that this will give them an advantage over their opponent. While gradual weight loss through sound nutritional and weight loss strategies to achieve an increase in the lean to fat ratio is justified, the use of crash weight reduction methods to achieve competitive weight will in many cases have a harmful effect not only on health but also on performance.

Methods Used to Make Weight

The most common methods of making weight are to increase the level of training, cut back calories and restrict fluid intake. Cutting out high fat snacks and eating smaller portions is sensible dieting but eating only one small meal a day, fasting completely, vomiting or taking diet pills is not.

Using simple dehydration techniques just prior to competition to lose the last remaining 0.5kg is acceptable (though the ideal is to reach competition weight without this being necessary) provided there is sufficient time to make up the fluid loss before the competition begins. Anything more drastic than this should be avoided. Some athletes can achieve large weight losses by staying in the sauna for several hours, working out in a heated gym in a rubber sweat suit, taking laxatives and diuretics (to increase the loss of body fluid as urine and faeces) and, of course, by not drinking any fluids, not even water.

How Performance and Health May be Affected

When food and fluid are severely restricted, water, fuel stores and some lean body mass will be lost. Some muscle strength may be lost and certainly endurance capacity will be reduced because there will be insufficient carbohydrate for glycogen synthesis to take place after training. At the next training session the athlete will feel tired and lethargic and put in a poor session. This could have both physiological and psychological effects on performance in the actual competition. Weight loss by dehydration can impair muscular performance and inhibit the sweating process which, in turn, increases the possibility of impairment in temperature regulation.

Once competition is over, there may be a great temptation to overeat resulting in

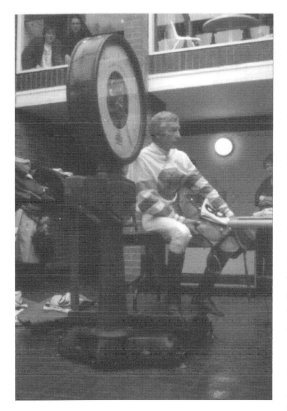

Lester Piggott in the weighing room before the second race of his comeback on Balasani, at Leicester races.

weight gain. This pattern of weight loss and regain is often repeated throughout the competitive season. Repeated weight cycling may increase the difficulty with which weight is lost in subsequent cycles.

Living, Training and Competition Weight

An athlete competing in a weight-sensitive sport should have his or her minimal weight estimated, by measuring body fat and calculating how much fat can be lost without affecting health or performance. This should be done by an exercise physiologist or sports dietitian who is qualified to take body fat

measurements, for example by using skinfold calipers. The difference between the present weight and minimal weight is the maximum amount of weight that can safely be lost.

An athlete must also identify his or her training weight band, which is the range of weights that can be maintained without too much difficulty during training, and his or her living weight band. This is the range of weights which may be reached when training eases up and the athlete lives normally, eating and drinking without restrictions. The greater the weight gain in the off-season, the more weight will have to be lost once training begins. By setting an upper limit to the living band and keeping a regular check during this time, a certain amount of damage limitation can be achieved. Ideally, athletes should train not more than 2kg away from their competition weight.

Making Competition Weight

A loss of 0.5kg through sweating out can be made up by drinking 500ml of an isotonic sports drink immediately after weighing-in but losing much more could mean total rehydration is not achieved before the competition begins. This should be borne in mind as the competition approaches.

To arrive at the right weight, or certainly very close to it, on the day before weighing-in, athletes may need to restrict fat intake more and more in the lead up to the competition. For example, this may be done by going from a thin spread of butter or margarine, to a thin scrape of low fat spread, and finally no spread at all. It is not a good idea to cut back on everything too early. Something should be kept in reserve for the final stages, in case things do not quite go to plan.

As training tapers down towards competition, portion sizes will need to be reduced and the actual content adjusted to provide more carbohydrate and less fat. Pasta with a little meat and tomato sauce with cheese becomes pasta with tomato sauce and a sprinkling of cheese, and then becomes pasta with enough tomato sauce to make the pasta palatable.

A regular check on body weight must be kept and food intake cut back accordingly. It often helps to keep a diary of food intake, fluid intake and body weight. Many athletes take a simple multivitamin and mineral supplement as an insurance policy (*see* Chapter 4).

When it comes to the countdown before the event, athletes still need to maintain their carbohydrate and fluid intake. If they have been refuelling correctly in the weeks leading up to competition, having their usual high carbohydrate meal the night before (portions according to energy output) will just keep the status quo as far as weight is concerned; in other words, it will not lead to a weight increase.

CHAPTER 7

Nutritional Ergogenic Aids

Athletes have experimented from ancient times to present day with pills and potions in the belief and hope that they will improve or optimize performance. At various levels of competition, athletes are so similar in ability that medals are won by millimetres or milliseconds. The ancient Greeks reportedly used stimulants to improve performance and the Aztecs claimed that eating hearts from human sacrifices had a beneficial effect on performance. Brandy and cocaine mixtures were supposedly favoured by boxers in the early 1900s, and in 1904 the English-born American Tom Hicks won the Olympic Marathon after being given a mixture of egg white, sulphate of strychnine, a stimulant and several sips of brandy.

Today, the favourites include creatine, carnitine, bicarbonate, caffeine, HMB and glutamine. Many athletes have used supplements containing Chinese herbs in an effort to improve performance.

NUTRITIONAL SUPPLEMENT OR ERGOGENIC AID?

Ergogenic comes from the Greek words *ergon* (work) and *gennan* (to produce) meaning work producing or work enhancing and therefore claiming to improve performance. Nutritional supplements are used to compensate for a less than adequate diet or lifestyle or to meet unusual or heavy demands of training or competition. These might include the use of a multivitamin and mineral supplement, an isotonic sports drink or a carbohydrate powder. The use and potential benefits of nutritional supplements have been covered in other chapters.

The difference between these nutritional supplements and nutritional ergogenic aids is that supplements do not raise performance above expectations. A female athlete who is iron deficient will underperform and taking an iron supplement will improve her performance or maximize her potential. However a female athlete who derives all the iron she needs from her diet and has good iron status will gain no performance benefits by taking extra iron as a supplement. Nutritional supplements do not raise performance above expectations but nutritional ergogenic aids are used in the belief or hope that they will do just that.

EVALUATING NUTRITIONAL ERGOGENIC AIDS

The nutritional ergogenics market is enormous and a positive minefield for the competitive athlete. Before using any product, athletes need to know the efficacy of the product (does it work and is it suitable in terms of their particular type of training and sport?), if it is safe and if it is legal. Ideally, there should be research papers, review articles and experts available to answer these questions. However, elite athletes are always looking for the competitive edge.

They want to be using a product before anyone else, so published data is unlikely to be available. Once research papers have been published and the product is generally available, the extra advantage will have been lost.

For the vast majority of athletes, awareness of particular ergogenic aids will only become apparent once their usage is more widespread. Creatine, perhaps the most popular ergogenic aid, provides a good example of this. An elite group of athletes were using creatine prior to the Barcelona Olympic Games in 1992, although most research investigating its efficacy in certain types of exercise was not published until later. Now professional, elite, amateur and recreational athletes use creatine and there is certainly no shortage of papers and reports on the use of creatine by the sporting and exercising populations.

In December 2000, The American Dietetic

Guidelines for Evaluating the Claims of Ergogenic Aids

Evaluate the Scientific Validity of an Ergogenic Claim by a Particular Supplement.
Does the amount and the form of the active ingredient claimed to be present in the supplement match that used in the scientific studies on this ergogenic aid?

Does the claim made by the manufacturer of the product match the science of nutrition and exercise as you know it?
Does the ergogenic claim make sense for the sport for which the claim is made?

Evaluate the Quality of the Supportive Evidence for Using the Ergogenic Aid.
What evidence is given for using the ergogenic aid (testimonial versus scientific study?)

What is the quality of the science?

What is the reputation of the author and the journal in which the research is published? Was the research sponsored by the manufacturer?

Does the experimental design meet the following criteria?
• hypothesis driven;
• double-blind placebo controlled;
• adequate and appropriate controls used; and
• appropriate dose of the ergogenic substance/placebo used?

What research methods were used and do they answer the questions asked? Are the methods clearly presented so the study results could be reproduced?

Are the methods clearly presented in an unbiased manner with appropriate statistical procedures, limitations addressed, and adverse events noted? Are the results physiologically feasible and do the conclusions follow from the data?

Evaluate the Safety and Legality of the Ergogenic Aid.
Is the product safe?

Will its use compromise the health of a person?

Does the product contain toxic or unknown substances or substances that alter nutrient metabolism?

Is the substance contraindicated in people with a particular health problem?

Will use of the product preclude other important elements in performance? For example, does the product claim to replace food or good training practices?

Is the product illegal or banned by any athletic organizations?

Permission to reproduce this section of the position statement has been obtained from the American Dietetic Association.

J. Am. Diet. Assoc (2000), Vol. 12, pp. 1543–56.

Association, Dietitians of Canada and the American College of Sports Medicine published a 'Joint Position Statement on Nutrition and Athletic Performance' which included guidelines for evaluating the claims of ergogenic aids (*Med. Sci. Sports Exerc.* Vol. 32, No. 12, pp. 2130–45; *J Am. Diet. Assoc.* (2000) Vol. 12, pp. 1543–56; *Diet of Canada* Vol. 61, pp 176–92).

Evaluating a Product

In the end the decision to use an ergogenic aid is down to the individual athlete, but that decision must be made only when a number of key questions have been answered. Using creatine as an example, the following shows how athletes could evaluate a potential ergogenic aid for themselves.

CREATINE SUPPLEMENTATION

First the background on creatine. It is a naturally occurring compound found in considerable amounts within meat and fish. Most of the body's stores of creatine are found in the skeletal muscle. In normal healthy individuals, muscle creatine degrades at the rate of 2g per day to creatinine which passes freely into the circulation and is excreted by the kidneys. The diet supplies about 1g per day for meat-eating individuals and the remainder is synthesized from amino acids to maintain the balance. Vegetarians obtain no creatine from the diet and the body therefore has to manufacture the entire requirement. There is some evidence that the body creatine stores are lower in vegetarians than in meat eaters.

Does Creatine Supplementation Work?

What is the available scientific information about the use of creatine and does it work in sport or training?

A search of the literature reveals that creatine appears to achieve its ergogenic effect by increasing pre-exercise muscle creatine phosphate availability and creatine phosphate re-synthesis during recovery. Scientifically, this makes sense. It is likely in the short-term to be of greatest benefit to those involved in repeated bouts of maximal exercise, as there is consistent evidence to show that using it improves recovery between each bout. Most studies show that increasing the amount of creatine in the muscles does not improve performance of the first bout or a single sprint, nor does it appear to have a beneficial effect in aerobic or endurance sports. Again most studies have been carried out using the dosages recommended by manufacturers. (There are manufacturers which advocate the use of higher doses although there are no scientific grounds for this.)

Some athletes have found no benefit from using creatine supplementation in the correct way for the right kind of exercise. Again turning to reputable research papers, it is possible to find a scientific explanation for this. Creatine is transported to the muscle by a membrane spanning protein. Sodium is also important for this process. Studies have shown that there is improved uptake if creatine is ingested with carbohydrate. This elevates insulin and stimulates the sodium pump action thus improving creatine transport. Athletes who initially did not respond to creatine supplementation found that by taking creatine with carbohydrate they too experienced benefits. So a search through current literature shows that creatine supplementation is based on valid scientific principles and could help certain athlete populations.

Is it Legal?

No athlete wants to be banned from his or her sport. An athlete must be absolutely sure that the product does not contain an ingredient that contravenes doping regulations. This may not be so simple to find out, as those athletes who have tested positive for nandrolone have found to their cost. The benefits of creatine are achieved by following a loading procedure and then dropping down to a daily low dose to ensure the raised level of creatine in the muscles is maintained. If an athlete decides to use creatine, it makes sense to buy a product that allows them to follow this procedure of loading followed by maintenance, in other words pure creatine monohydrate. Creatine is not a banned substance by any international sporting federation.

Is it Safe?

Creatine is a low molecular weight compound and its removal by the kidneys is achieved by diffusion, which is a non-energy dependent process. Ingestion of 20g per day for five days (the standard loading technique) is therefore considered to be of minimal risk to normal healthy individuals. Ingestion of larger doses is a waste of money. There is at the moment no evidence linking creatine supplementation with kidney damage in healthy individuals.

Creatine supplementation does cause an increase in urinary creatine and creatinine excretion (often used as an indicator of kidney failure). However this increase correlates well with the increase in muscle creatine observed during supplementation and reflects the increased rate of muscle creatine degradation to creatinine rather than any abnormality of renal function. It should be stressed that the long-term health risks of chronic ingestion of large amounts of creatine are at the moment unknown. However, with respect to the more common loading regime of 20g per day for five days, full haematological and clinical chemistry screening has been carried out before and after supplementation and no adverse effects have been recorded.

Creatine loading is associated with some immediate weight gain of 1 to 2kg. This is probably due to the retention of fluid with creatine in the muscle cell. Longer-term weight gains are probably due to increases in lean body mass as the athlete is able to train harder. There are numerous anecdotal reports of creatine supplementation causing muscle cramps and gastro-intestinal problems but no real definitive evidence of adverse effects in normal healthy adults.

Is it Being Used Correctly?

Studies have shown that 20g per day for five days (as 5g creatine dissolved in approximately 250ml of drink four times a day) can increase the body's creatine store which can, in some situations, improve performance. The majority of the initial studies have used this loading technique. More recently it has been shown that ingesting 95g of carbohydrate (such as Lucozade, but not Lucozade Sport) with 5g creatine leads to a 60 per cent increase in intra-cellular creatine. Taking creatine in such a way probably reduces the loading time necessary to ensure creatine stores will be saturated, from five to two days.

Once maximal concentrations of creatine are reached, the concentration drops off very slowly over four weeks. However, muscle creatine stores can be maintained by the use of a maintenance dose of 2g per day. Low doses (3g per day) on their own appear to be less effective, certainly over the short-term (fourteen days) though some researchers have suggested that elevated muscle creatine levels can be reached with low doses over a period of twenty-eight days.

THE BOTTOM LINE

Most nutritional ergogenic aids fall into one of the following categories:

- Those that perform as claimed (for example creatine, caffeine, bicarbonate).
- Those that may perform as claimed but more scientific evidence is needed (for example beta-hydroxy-beta-methyl-butyrate or HMB, glutamine and glucosamine).
- Those that do not perform as claimed (for example chromium picolinate, carnitine, coenzyme Q10).
- Those that are banned by national and international sporting organisations (for example supplements containing ephedra, androstenedione, 19-norandrostenedione and 19-norandrostenediol).

The ethical issue of using performance-enhancing supplements which are not banned is one that athletes must resolve for themselves. Before that decision is made, the athlete must have evaluated the product and discussed its use with a qualified (and understanding) sports doctor, sports scientist or sports dietitian/nutritionist. Many nutritional supplements and some nutritional ergogenic aids do have a role to play in helping athletes to meet their ultimate goals: to improve performance, remain fit, healthy and injury-free, recover from injury or illness quickly and to maintain their 'best' weight or body composition. However it must be remembered they are no substitute for, only a supplement to:

- A well-planned training programme.
- Adequate rest and recovery.
- Well-planned mental preparation.
- The right equipment.
- The optimal diet for training and competition.

No attempt has been made to evaluate the plethora of ergogenic aids that are marketed. New ones will continue to appear, some with but most without any scientific basis or evaluation. More information on this subject can be found in Melvin H Williams, *The ergogenics edge: pushing the limits of sports performance* (Human Kinetics, 1998) (ISBN 0-88011-545-9).

To access scientific publications on this subject, contact the National Sports Medicine Institute library (*see* Appendix IV).

CHAPTER 8

The Young Athlete

The dietary requirements of children are different to those of adults. However those children who are involved in sport at a competitive level are set apart even from other children when considering the practical aspects of their diet. The underlining principles of the diet remain the same, but lifestyle and the demands of training together with the requirements of the sport itself will necessitate some dietary modifications.

The special nutritional concerns when working with children in sport are:

- energy requirement;
- carbohydrate intake;
- protein intake;
- vitamin and mineral intake;
- eating habits;
- weight control and body composition; and
- fluid replacement.

ENERGY REQUIREMENTS

Childhood and adolescence are times of rapid growth and development with parallel increases in nutritional requirements. Because of the demands of growth, children require a higher energy intake than adults in proportion to their weight. Absolute energy needs for growth are higher during adolescence than in childhood years.

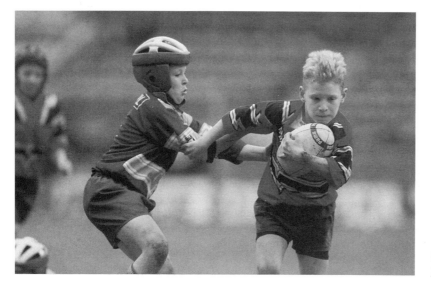

Children's Rugby League.

Estimated Average Requirements for Energy (EAR)		
Age	Males (kcal per day)	Females (kcal per day)
7 to 10 years	1,970	1,740
11 to 14 years	2,220	1,845
15 to 18 years	2,755	2,110

The energy requirement will also vary with the level of physical activity.

Poor energy intakes that do not match requirements over a significant period of time can result in growth retardation, delayed puberty, nutrient deficiencies such as iron deficiency anaemia, menstrual irregularities, poor bone health, increased incidence of injuries and increased risk of developing eating disorders.

ADEQUATE CARBOHYDRATE INTAKE

The benefits of high carbohydrate diets in enhancing performance are well documented. The dietary aim with young athletes is to get 55 per cent of total energy from carbohydrate,

Estimated Average Requirement for Energy for Children and Adolescents (10 to 18 years) According to Body Weight and Physical Activity Level (PAL)

Males

Body weight (kg)	BMR kcal/d	1.4	1.5	PAL 1.6	1.8	2.0
30	1,188	1,673	1,793	1,912	2,151	2,366
35	1,276	1,793	1,912	2,055	2,294	2,557
40	1,365	1,912	2,055	2,175	2,462	2,725
45	1,453	2,032	2,175	2,318	2,629	2,916
50	1,542	2,151	2,318	2,462	2,772	3,083
55	1,630	2,294	2,438	2,605	2,940	3,250
60	1,718	2,414	2,581	2,749	3,083	3,442
65	1,807	2,533	2,700	2,892	3,250	3,609

Females

Body weight (kg)	BMR kcal/d	1.4	1.5	PAL 1.6	1.8	2.0
30	1,095	1,530	1,649	1,745	1,960	2,200
35	1,162	1,625	1,745	1,864	2,079	2,318
40	1,228	1,721	1,840	1,960	2,200	2,462
45	1,295	1,816	1,936	2,079	2,342	2,581
50	1,362	1,912	2,032	2,175	2,462	2,725
55	1,429	2,008	2,151	2,294	2,581	2,868
60	1,496	2,103	2,247	2,390	2,700	2,988

(Source: Calculated from data published in Department of Health Report of Health and Social Subjects, No. 41 *Dietary reference values for food energy and nutrients for the United Kingdom: Report of the Panel on Dietary Reference Values, Committee on Medical Aspects of Food Policy* (HMSO, 1991).)

30 per cent total energy from fat and 15 per cent total energy from protein. These intakes in no way conflict with generally accepted healthy eating guidelines. This requires a certain degree of education and implementation, as there is no evidence that athletic youngsters are any better than non-athletic youngsters at eating more carbohydrate-rich foods and fewer fatty foods.

Young athletes need to be shown why this balance is so important (of course for health) but also for sporting performance. They need to develop a working knowledge of the best food sources and the relevant contributions made by starch and sugar to their overall carbohydrate intake. The need for good dental hygiene must also be emphasized. Getting the message across may not be the hardest part of the process but implementation may be harder. For example, no one has a greater need for food than an active, growing teenage athlete particularly one involved in a high-energy sport such as football. Meeting the needs of such a teenager may not be easy given financial, social and lifestyle constraints.

PROTEIN INTAKES

The protein needs of children and adolescents are higher than those of sedentary adults. As the protein requirements of adult athletes are higher than those of sedentary adults, it is possible that those of young athletes might also be higher than their less active peers. Protein intakes have to meet the requirements of growth, development and training. However there are no published studies of young athletes' protein requirements and specific recommendations cannot be made. Muscle growth comes from consuming a diet containing sufficient energy, protein and other essential nutrients, training. It also comes from physical maturity, the stage of development when hormones are released in sufficient amounts to stimulate muscle growth.

VITAMIN AND MINERAL INTAKES

Requirements for several vitamins are highest in the teenage years. Excessive consumption of sugary foods and drinks could lead to less than optimal intakes of some vitamins. There can be a risk of inadequate intake of vitamins if food intake is restricted, especially amongst those who chronically restrict energy intake in order to maintain a low body weight. Again education is the key, to show young athletes how to choose foods to give dietary quality as well as quantity. Vitamin supplementation may be useful in some situations. However the aim should be to meet all vitamin requirements by diet alone. Supplement usage can give the wrong message, encouraging young athletes not to bother with their diet and just rely on supplementation.

The minerals of particular concern are calcium and iron. The requirements for these minerals are high in childhood and adolescence (the need for calcium is greater during adolescence than at any other time) and inadequate intakes can affect both short-term and long-term health and sporting performance. Poor intakes can often be caused by misinformed advice (perhaps cutting out dairy produce or meat because of the fat content) or a lack of sound nutritional knowledge (for example by adopting a vegetarian lifestyle without a proper understanding of how to replace the nutrients normally obtained from eating meat). As with vitamins, restricted food intake will affect the intake of minerals.

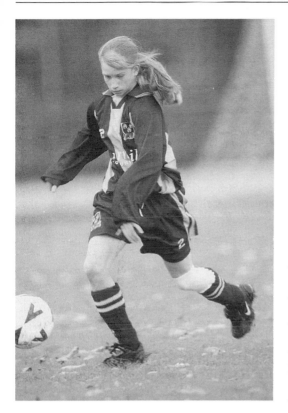

Sam Bartley of Shrewsbury Town Women's Football Club.

EATING HABITS

Adolescence, a period of rapid physical growth and change, is also a period of emotional and psychological change, when the independent character of the individual is established. There is a tendency to reject convention and to exert independence by making individual choices. Friends start to have more influence than parents do in areas such as eating behaviour and patterns. Meals may be missed (particularly breakfast), there may be frequent snacking, fast and take-away foods may make up a large proportion of total food intake, unconventional meals may be enjoyed and, of course, unnecessary dieting may be under-

taken or become extreme. Linking a healthy diet with improved sporting performance can be used as a strong motivator for positive change.

WEIGHT CONTROL AND BODY COMPOSITION

Growth and development during childhood and adolescence is normal and desirable but some children and teenagers become very susceptible to weight control problems during this period. Young sportsmen often seek advice about 'bulking up' while young sportswomen often face difficult problems and choices in trying to juggle growth, strength, weight and optimal body fat. The post-pubertal female gains fat naturally, while her sport may demand unnatural thinness. Some females believe weight loss will enhance performance. It may do so initially, but weight loss can be carried too far, both in terms of health and performance. Where weight loss or gain is accepted as necessary this should be achieved safely, legally and with minimum fuss with the help of a sports dietitian or sports nutritionist.

FLUID REPLACEMENT

Young sportspeople are high risk candidates for dehydration because they are less efficient at thermoregulation and more susceptible to heat stress. Children particularly are at a greater risk of dehydration because they are poor at coping with extremes of temperature, sweat less, get hotter during exercise, have a lower heart output and have a greater surface area for their weight.

Certain conditions can make the situation worse; for example the protective clothing required in some sports can reduce the ability to cool down. Young swimmers are wet anyway and often do not realize how much body fluid they are losing. The temperature and humidity of many swimming pools does not help the situation.

Young sports people need to be educated in how they can adequately maintain their own hydration, in other words to know what and when to drink. Coaches, teachers and parents must play their part too, for example checking at the start of every training session that each child has a drinks bottle with an appropriate fluid in it. Children do not instinctively or voluntarily replenish fluid losses during exercise and yet they are at greater risk of dehydration than adults are. It is therefore important that children are reminded to drink to a schedule (every 15 to 20 minutes) during training or exercise.

Children should be allowed to drink until they feel their thirst is satisfied but then encouraged to drink some more because their thirst mechanism is poorly developed. Young athletes who are particularly irritable at the end of a training session should be carefully monitored to assess how much fluid they are habitually drinking. Water is an acceptable drink, especially when there is nothing else available but it does not provide energy, is less appealing than a flavoured drink (so less is drunk) and is less effective at maintaining hydration than a properly formulated sports drink.

CHAPTER 9

The Female Athlete

The benefits of regular exercise are well documented but it is still possible to have too much of a good thing. There is increasing concern about the medical problems that are becoming more and more prevalent amongst the athletic female population. The female athlete who pushes herself to the limits either in her chosen sport or in a demanding exercise regime may be at risk of developing what is known as the 'female triad'. Intensive training programmes need to be sustained by a diet that provides energy, nutrients and fluid in the required amounts for the athlete. Unfortunately many female athletes and active women believe that cutting back food intake and losing weight will improve performance

and appearance. For some athletes a reduction in body fat may well lead to improved performances but this can be carried too far, resulting not only in a loss of performance but also in serious health consequences.

THE FEMALE TRIAD

The female triad describes three interrelated conditions: disordered eating, amenorrhoea (no periods) and bone loss, which brings a potential risk of developing premature osteoporosis (brittle bone disease). Disordered eating describes a range of abnormal patterns of eating, of which the most common among female

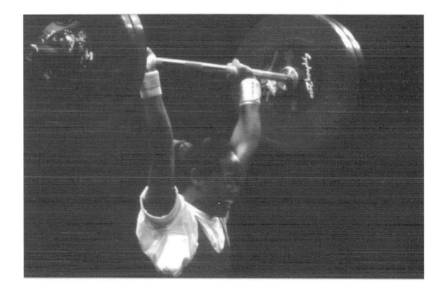

Indonesia's Binti Winarni Slamet lifts for a Bronze medal.

athletes are *anorexia nervosa* and *bulimia nervosa*. Such conditions may start with avoidance of certain foods, restriction of food intake to one meal a day or with an obsession about fat in food and a resulting exclusion of foods from the diet that are above a particular fat content.

Diagnostic criteria, physical symptoms and psychological and behavioural characteristics of athletes with these conditions are clearly identified. Many of these symptoms can be picked up by physiotherapists and doctors working with athletes while other warning signs might be noticed by team or squad members. Eating disorders appear to be more common amongst those involved in gymnastics, distance running, diving, ballet, figure skating and weight category sports, although vulnerable females from any sport may present. Male athletes with eating disorders are less common, although the problem is certainly observed among wrestlers, boxers and jockeys.

HEALTH IMPLICATIONS OF EATING DISORDERS

Eating disorders may cause serious health problems and can even result in death. In

---

Signs of Anorexia Nervosa

Physical Signs
Severe weight loss.
Irregular or no periods.
Difficulty in sleeping.
Frequent dizzy spells.
Complains of stomach pains, constipation or feelings of bloatedness.
Growth of downy hair on face, legs and arms.
Complains of feeling the cold.

Psychological Signs
Athlete insists she is fat when obviously underweight.
Athlete is irritable.
Athlete sets unreasonably high standards.
Athlete becomes obsessed with training hard and longer.
Athlete prefers to run alone.
Athlete is more aware of food and calories.

Behavioural Signs
Athlete starts exercising excessively.
Others suspect she is lying about eating.
Athlete refuses to eat in company.
Athlete willingly cooks and provides food for others.

Signs of Bulimia Nervosa

Physical Signs
Abrasions on the back of the knuckles from inducing vomiting.
Athlete suffers frequent dehydration even when not training or competing.
Athlete has dental and gum problems.
Athlete has extreme weight fluctuations.
Athlete reports menstrual irregularities.
Athlete complains about muscle cramps and weakness.
Athlete has swollen salivary glands at the side of the face.

Psychological Signs
Athlete suffers depression.
Athlete becomes increasingly self-critical, especially about her body and performance.
Athlete has noticeable mood swings.

Behavioural Signs
Athlete eats large quantities of food and is sick after meals.
Athlete starts diets which are unnecessary for appearance, health or performance.
Athlete visits the toilet or 'disappears' after eating.
Athlete uses laxatives and/or diuretics.
Athlete steals food and laxatives.
Athlete becomes secretive and lies about eating.

anorexia nervosa, health problems occur simply due to starvation but in bulimia nervosa they are the result of binge eating and purging. Loss of fluid and electrolytes can lead to dehydration and electrolyte abnormalities which in turn affect coordination, balance and muscle function.

MENSTRUAL IRREGULARITIES

Female athletes who undergo hard training often find that their periods stop or at least that their menstrual cycle becomes irregular. This is more likely to happen as the training intensity increases. For instance, loss of periods (amenorrhoea) is much more common in women running 80 miles a week compared with those who run only 20 miles a week. The prevalence of menstrual dysfunction appears to be significantly higher among athletes who compete in sports that demand leanness or where an athlete must compete at a specific weight than amongst those who compete in sports where these factors are of less importance.

Many female athletes are at the same time restricting energy intake in an attempt to lose weight or maintain a low body weight and this contributes to the development of amenorrhoea. The combination of energy restriction and increased energy output leads to major changes in body composition, in particular to a reduction of body fat. Body fat can fall to very low levels, which are too low to support a pregnancy, so as a protection against conception periods stop temporarily. Thus a reduction in body fat composition is linked to amenorrhoea or to irregularities of the menstrual cycle (oligomenorrhoea).

Bone Loss

Concern about the clinical implications of amenorrhoea initially centred on the loss of reproductive function but more recently has switched to the immediate and potential long-term effects of low levels of oestrogen on bone mass. Amenorrhoeic athletes with low body fat levels and low levels of circulating oestrogen behave rather like post-menopausal women. They experience accelerated bone loss resulting in reduced bone density and this in turn puts them at greater risk of suffering a traumatic or stress fracture. Even if bone density does not fall so low that stress fractures occur, there is a long-term health concern. Young women who are losing bone when they should still be accumulating it will have a lower peak bone mass in mid-adulthood and this will inevitably increase the risk of osteoporosis and bone fractures in late adulthood.

Treatment of Amenorrhoea

Bone loss can occur quickly in the young female athlete who has stopped having periods and athletes should be encouraged to seek treatment as soon as possible. Treatment of amenorrhoea aims to prevent bone loss and to re-establish a normal menstrual cycle. The latter can take time, which may be too slow to minimize the effect on the athlete's bones, particularly if she has been amenorrhoeic for some time. In this case the likely treatment to be suggested will be the use of hormone therapy to boost the level of circulating oestrogen. Changes in lifestyle will take longer and will of course need the cooperation of the athlete.

A female athlete who appears to be in danger of developing the female triad should be encouraged to decrease training activity by 10 to 20 per cent and increase energy intake, in order to achieve a weight gain of 2 to 3 per cent of her current body weight. Calcium intake should be increased to 1,500mg per day, and resistance training used to boost muscle strength and help bone mineralization. The athlete should be strongly encouraged to consult a sports dietitian.

Dietary Counselling

This is just one facet of the treatment, which invariably also involves medical and psychological treatment. The aim is not to prescribe yet another diet but to guide the athlete back to eating in a normal and relaxed way with sufficient flexibility to adapt to various social situations such as eating in a restaurant or with friends. Accurate information and the safety and control that meal plans can afford will help the athlete to reduce her apprehension about, and resistance to, changing her eating patterns.

Athletes with eating disorders often believe they are very knowledgeable about nutrition when in fact they are not. They know all about calories and the fat content of food but little about the nutritional worth of foods or what is meant by a balanced diet or normal eating. They are often experts in deception and manipulation and can sense if anyone involved in their treatment or counselling is vulnerable or inexperienced. They are capable of exploiting perceived weaknesses by lying, making the counsellor feel inadequate or by arousing conflict between other professionals involved. The ideal approach is therefore to be confident, sympathetic, understanding but with an element of firmness.

A FINAL WORD

Athletes, coaches and teachers, parents, sports science and sports medicine staff and administrators in sport should consider the following points when working with female athletes.

Sports participation should be promoted for physical and mental health and healthy eating habits go hand in hand with good performance (eat well, perform better). Poor diet and eating habits do not. Body weight and body composition should be de-emphasized as a major factor in measuring performance and myths that being thin improves performance should be dispelled (too thin to win).

The natural changes that occur at puberty must be acknowledged and not fought against. Athletes should be encouraged to monitor their menstrual cycle and report any changes to a person in authority who they can trust and who will know any action to take. This might be a parent, coach, team doctor, sports dietitian or physiotherapist.

The whole subject of the female athlete triad is enormously sensitive and complex both in terms of aetiology (cause), diagnosis and treatment. It is a subject too big to cover in any depth in this book. Instead the aim of the author has been to help athletes, parents and all those involved in sport be more aware of the condition and its symptoms, and to give some contact details where support and further information can be obtained. A series of three leaflets (*Eating Disorders – an athlete's guide, Eating Disorders – a coach's guide* and *Eating Disorders – a guide for friends and relatives*) can be obtained by sending a stamped addressed A5 envelope to DISEN or UK Athletics (*see* Appendix IV).

CHAPTER 10

The Older Athlete

The diet for the older athlete is no different from that recommended for the younger athlete. The knowledge that the diet meets healthy eating guidelines and therefore may help in reducing the risk of heart disease, stroke and some forms of cancer will undoubtedly be of more interest to the older athlete.

A master athlete who trains regularly will benefit from a high carbohydrate, low fat diet. A high fibre intake, achieved by choosing more whole grain carbohydrate foods can help to relieve constipation, which is a common problem for older people. Vitamin requirements do not change with age but as active older people have a greater energy requirement than their sedentary friends, a greater food intake should supply all the vitamins and minerals that are needed. Sedentary individuals may not meet their vitamin requirements or, alternatively, they may eat enough to meet vitamin requirements but more than they need to meet their energy requirement with the result that weight increases gradually with increasing age. However there are some aspects of the diet that the older athlete does need to address specifically.

KEEPING HYDRATED

Ageing has traditionally been associated with a reduction in tolerance to heat but it is now understood that though age does play a part, poor physical fitness, disease processes and lack of acclimatization are more significant. Older people seem less efficient at losing heat through sweating, as the sweat response to exercise is slower and reduced. However with physical training this can be improved. Older people are also less aware of the sensations of thirst and ageing athletes competing in hot, dry conditions could be significantly dehydrated before the desire to drink kicks in.

To minimize dehydration and prevent heat-related problems when training or competing in the heat, older athletes should ensure full hydration before the start of the event and should be careful to replace fluids as soon as possible into the event rather than waiting until a sensation of thirst is felt. After the event, the athlete should continue drinking until full hydration status has been restored.

It is advisable to remain in the shade as much as possible and wear light coloured clothing including a protective hat if this is feasible and permitted (for example during an 18 hole round of golf).

The older athlete should aim to take exercise when the sun is less intense (before 10am and after 4pm if possible). It is sensible to ensure optimal fitness level and not to compete if fitness level is significantly reduced. All athletes should be aware of the warning signs of heat stress: muscle cramps, dizziness, cool dry skin, quickening pulse, nausea, excessive thirst and fatigue.

EXERCISE IN THE COLD

Older athletes are at greater risk of frostbite because their awareness of the degree of cold may be reduced. With ageing there is a gradual reduction in the adipose tissue under the skin and this reduces the insulation which is afforded to more well-padded individuals. If there is any narrowing of the arteries (athero-sclerosis) present this will reduce the flow of warm blood to the peripheral tissues that are being cooled down by the cold environmental temperature.

EXERCISE AT ALTITUDE

Many sporting activities enjoyed by older people take place at altitude, such as hiking, climbing, running and skiing. On the plus side, altitude sickness appears to be less severe with age, regardless of the speed of ascent. On the negative side, older athletes will have more problems obtaining enough oxygen, partly because less oxygen is available from the atmosphere but also because the ageing process means less is delivered to the working muscles. However, as with hydration, an individual's ability to tolerate altitude is dependent more on health and fitness than on age.

INJURIES

The ageing athlete is more vulnerable to injury as tendons and muscles stiffen, rate of tissue repair slows, joints become less supple and flexible and bone mass is lost. The injured older athlete also seems to be at greater risk of developing complications such as infections. Diet plays a part in the healing processes and the ageing athlete must ensure that the diet provides all the nutrients important to this process (*see* Chapter 12).

CHAPTER 11

The Vegetarian Athlete

The term 'vegetarian' can embrace a whole variety of diets.

- Semi- or demi-vegetarians avoid only red meat but eat poultry, fish, dairy foods and eggs.
- Pesco-vegetarians eat dairy foods, eggs and fish but no other animal flesh.
- Lacto-ovo-vegetarians eat dairy products and eggs but no animal flesh.
- Lacto-vegetarians eat dairy foods but no eggs or animal flesh.
- Ovo-vegetarians eat eggs but no dairy foods or animal flesh.
- Vegans avoid all animal products in their diets.

All the nutrients needed to support training and competition and to maintain health can be obtained from vegetarian food sources. However it is not just a simple case of cutting out meat and eating a few more vegetables. The foods selected to make up a vegetarian diet must provide all the nutrients that would otherwise have been obtained from animal sources.

A vegetarian diet should contain plenty of cereal-based foods (bread, pasta, rice and breakfast cereals), fruit and vegetables and beans, peas and lentils. This type of diet is not only good news in terms of long-term health, helping to prevent heart disease and certain forms of cancer, but it can also provide significant amounts of the carbohydrate so essential in an athlete's diet. One note of caution: vegetarians who eat dairy products need to be careful that they do not eat too much fat (and particularly saturated fat). Milk, cheese and yoghurts should all be included but choices must be made from the large range of low fat or reduced fat dairy products available.

Generally, proteins from animal sources provide all the eight essential amino acids needed by children and adults while vegetable sources tend to be low in one or more of these essential amino acids. To get enough of all the essential amino acids, vegetarians who do not eat dairy foods or eggs need to eat a wide range of vegetable sources of protein, particularly legumes (peas, beans and lentils), grains and seeds. In the past such vegetarians were recommended to plan each meal so that the amino acids in the different proteins complemented each other. Nowadays this is considered unnecessary as long as the diet contains plenty of variety on a daily basis.

WHAT COULD BE MISSING IN A VEGETARIAN DIET?

Athletes who eat fish and poultry really have nothing to worry about. Lacto-ovo vegetarians should still find it fairly easy to get all the essential nutrients, while being careful to choose low fat options as depending too heavily on milk, cheese and eggs for the main protein source of the diet could lead to an unnecessarily high fat intake. Those athletes who avoid all flesh, including red meat, poultry and fish need to do some careful planning, particularly to make sure the diet contains sufficient iron, zinc and the essential fatty acids present in oily fish. A vegan will have to take extra time to plan meals and snacks and may even need to take a vitamin supplement. Vitamin B_{12} is normally found only in animal foods such as meat, fish, eggs and dairy products or in foods fortified with this vitamin (such as breakfast cereals and some soya milks). If these foods are not consumed, a supplement would normally be recommended.

Dairy products are normally the main source of calcium in the diet. If these foods are excluded from the diet an alternative dietary sources of calcium must be found. Those who experience difficulty in meeting their requirement from food alone may need to take a dietary supplement of calcium. Athletes who are concerned that this applies to them should arrange for their diet to be checked by their general practitioner, sports doctor or sports dietitian. Iron from vegetable sources is not absorbed as well as that from animal sources. It is also present in much smaller amounts compared with the amounts in meat. Eating foods that contain vitamin C together with any iron-containing food will improve absorption; for example drinking orange juice with fortified breakfast cereal or adding tomatoes to sandwiches. (*See* Chapter 4 for more information about calcium and iron in the diet.)

How to Meet Nutrient Needs

Protein

Eat plenty of beans, peas and lentils, grains and seeds.

Use Quorn and tofu as meat replacements in meals such as meat-free Bolognese, stir-frys and kebabs.

Combine milk or eggs with these foods to get the right balance of protein, for example cheese or egg sandwiches, macaroni cheese, breakfast cereal with milk or yoghurt and milk puddings.

Combine cereals with peas, beans and lentils, for example baked beans on toast, lentil curry and rice, vegetarian chilli with rice, pasta and mixed bean salad.

Some ready-made products will be suitable, convenient ways to build up the diet (especially when there are constraints on time).

Calcium

Include dairy products, dark green leafy vegetables, fortified soya milk, pulses, peanuts (peanut butter), almonds and seeds.

Iron

Include peas, beans and lentils, dark green leafy vegetables, dried fruits, fortified breakfast cereals and breads.

Vitamin B_{12}

Include dairy products, eggs, fermented soya products and vitamin B_{12} fortified foods and supplements.

CHAPTER 12

The Injured Athlete

All those who train, compete or work out regularly dread the injury or illness that prevents them from exercising and will search for anything that will speed up recovery and help them back to full fitness. Diet has a role to play in both prevention and recovery from injury and illness.

INJURY PREVENTION

Some years ago, a survey of recreational and competitive downhill skiers in Holland found that many skiers pointed out that towards the end of the day they were too tired to avoid a fall that led to an injury. It is difficult to show a cause and effect relationship between fatigue and injury but there is evidence that suggests an association. Fatigued individuals are vulnerable to injury; in fact they are almost waiting for an accident to happen. More recently a study of injury prevention strategies in professional footballers identified a lack of awareness of the benefits of carbohydrate intake before and after training and matches, along with the importance of the use of shin pads, cooling down after training and matches, and flexibility work.

Depleted muscle glycogen stores are associated with fatigue. It is therefore important to start each exercise session with full stores of muscle glycogen in order to avoid or at least

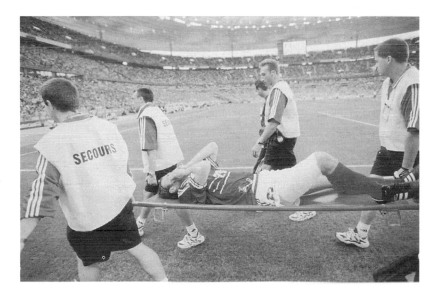

France's Christophe Dugarry is carried off after sustaining an injury, putting him out for the rest of the 1998 World Cup.

delay severe depletion until as late as possible into the session. Muscle protein is broken down in both strength and endurance training. To compensate, protein synthesis is increased post-exercise. If the diet contains insufficient protein, there is a risk that strength will be lost, another potential cause of injury.

Calcium is vital for maintaining bone mass. Although by no means the only factor, a poor calcium intake has been linked to lower bone mineral density, a potential cause of stress fractures. Poor iron status can also have an adverse effect. Low ferritin levels lead to a decreased delivery of oxygen to the muscles so that muscles become fatigued more easily.

Exercise increases the production of free radicals which may be the cause of muscle damage, soreness and inflammation often experienced after strenuous exercise. Exercise stimulates the body's natural defence mechanisms to produce antioxidants to help neutralize the free radicals. Although there is continuing debate as to the benefit of taking antioxidant supplements, there is no disagreement that a regular intake of fruit and vegetables is beneficial.

A dehydrated body fatigues quickly, not only physically but also mentally. Injuries through mental tiredness will occur because of lapses in concentration, errors, slowed reaction time and task inaccuracies. Practical ways of addressing all these aspects of the diet have been dealt with in previous chapters.

DIET AND THE HEALING PROCESS

It has long been known that adequate amounts of protein, vitamins and minerals are needed for the healing process and that inadequate amounts can delay the process or lead to poor healing.

It is important to take into account changes in energy requirements, particularly if an extended lay-off is envisaged. Injured athletes may not automatically reduce their food intake to match the drop in physical activity level. The resulting increase in body fat may slow the process of rehabilitation and return to form. Muscle mass will be lost if weights sessions have to be stopped or if surgery requires parts of the body to be immobilized. Bulking-up diets may be needed at some stages during the rehabilitation programme (*see* Chapter 6).

Although there may be a need to reduce energy intake, it is also important to ensure adequate amounts of protein, iron, zinc, calcium and vitamin C are consumed as these all have a part to play in the healing process. Most athletes will find they need to reduce their intake of carbohydrate because their requirements are lower, and also in order to reduce the overall energy intake. Protein intake should not be reduced but neither should fat intake be increased.

It may be difficult for some athletes to maintain their diet while they are injured. Getting to the supermarket may be difficult because of reduced mobility or cooking may be difficult: trying to open a can with one hand can send frustration levels soaring. Fractured jaws can pose a problem with the actual mechanism of eating. However, a sports dietitian will be able to offer advice to ensure the diet contains the correct amounts of the nutrients essential for healing and will be able to ensure that the advice is practical for the athlete's lifestyle and injury.

Time out through injury can provide an opportunity for the athlete to work with a sports dietitian not only on rehabilitation but also on building up a picture of the best diet when back to full training. This can provide a positive goal during the injury phase.

André Agassi receives treatment from the Queen's Club physio for an injury to his back.

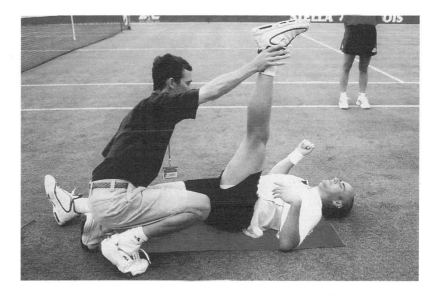

WHAT ABOUT SUPPLEMENTS?

Eating five portions of fruit and vegetables a day will help to ensure a good intake of anti oxidant nutrients and phytochemicals. For those athletes who genuinely struggle to eat sufficient fruit and vegetables, an antioxidant supplement would be a sensible precaution.

Some sports doctors and physiotherapists have advised the use of glucosamine, an amino acid which is needed by chrondrocytes (cells that make up cartilage) to function properly. Although research to date is scanty it is possible that glucosamine may be helpful in speeding up the healing of injured joints. Anecdotal evidence is not lacking!

Regular use of cod liver oil (which contains high levels of the essential omega-3 fatty acids) also appears to help keep joints supple and flexible and, again, there is some evidence that it helps in reducing inflammation and may even help to protect cartilage from wear and tear. Although there is limited research into the claimed benefits, use of cod liver oil has certainly stood the test of time. Another case, perhaps, of 'Granny knows best'.

THE STITCH

The cause of the stitch is still not totally understood. It may be due to lack of oxygen as blood flow is diverted from non-exercising areas to the muscles. Equally it may be due to dehydration or even micronutrient im-balance. More recently it has been suggested that it could be caused by tugging of the gut on ligaments connecting the gut to the diaphragm.

Stitches seem to be less common amongst highly-trained athletes. There appears to be no link with food intake before exercise and many athletes believe that keeping well hydrated helps to prevent stitch development. To date, maintaining an adequate fluid intake appears to be the best advice to avoid a getting a stitch together with drinking small frequent amounts during exercise rather than large volumes less often. It is also sensible to avoid exercising straight after a meal or large drink if prone to stitches.

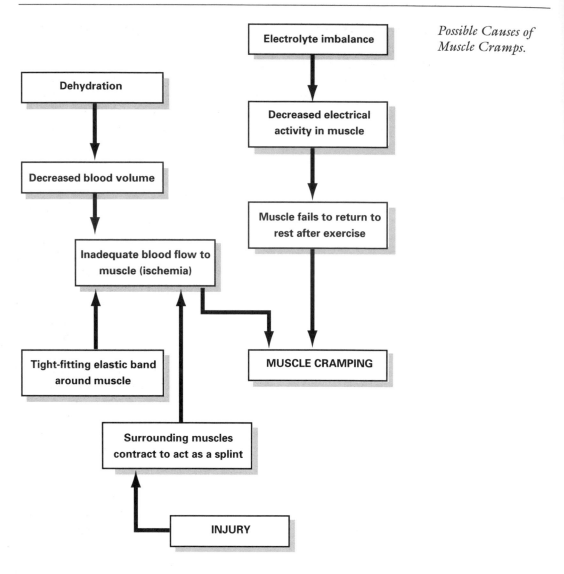

Possible Causes of Muscle Cramps.

MUSCLE CRAMPS

Like the stitch, the cause and prevention of cramps remains a puzzle. They seem more likely to appear when an athlete exercises to near exhaustion, is less well trained, becomes dehydrated or has an electrolyte imbalance. Electrolyte imbalance is often a result of drinking water during endurance and ultra-endurance exercise but with little or no electrolyte replacement.

Keeping up a good fluid intake seems to be the best advice in order to avoid cramp. Using a sports drink rather than water will help to maintain hydration and electrolyte balance. Addition of salt to food can be helpful, particularly when training or competing in the heat.

GASTRO-INTESTINAL PROBLEMS

Constipation is not a common problem amongst the athletic population, as one of the many benefits of regular exercise is a bowel that works well. For any athletes who do suffer from a sluggish bowel, the dietary advice is simple: increase the intake of fruit and vegetables, dietary fibre and fluids. A drink of warm water (if desired, flavoured with lemon) first thing in the morning may help.

On the other hand, diarrhoea or runner's trots, abdominal cramping, wind and heartburn are all common problems. The causes are numerous and invariably related to the food and fluid consumed before and during exercise.

Frequent digestive problems during or after running, for example, may be alleviated by switching training runs from morning to evening or vice versa. Avoid high fibre foods for twenty-four to thirty-six hours before a race and generally do not consume excessive amounts of fibre on a day-to-day basis (*see* Chapter 4). A warm drink or a bowl of hot cereal some hours before a long run can sometimes encourage the bowel to work in time. If possible try to have a bowel movement before exercise (this might eventually become a regular pre-exercise habit). Avoid beans, cabbage, broccoli and Brussels sprouts, particularly before a race, to reduce wind and bloating.

REDUCING THE RISK OF ILLNESS

Illnesses, particularly frequent or lingering ones can be a major source of disruption to training programmes. Although difficult to avoid there are measures an athlete can take to reduce the risk of catching an infection or at least lessening the severity once a cold, for example, is caught.

For colds and upper respiratory tract infections where the symptoms are all above the neck, light exercise will help speed recovery (low intensity for between five and seven days until symptoms disappear). Symptoms below the neck require complete rest and a visit to the doctor. Taking 500 to 1,000mg vitamin C per day immediately once cold symptoms appear may help to lessen the severity and possibly the duration of a cold. Taking large doses of vitamin C on a regular basis will not prevent a cold.

Exposure to infections can be reduced by being scrupulous about personal hygiene, for example washing hands after using the toilet and before preparing and eating food, avoiding sharing food, utensils and towels and avoiding close contact with anyone with an infection. Drinks bottles should never be shared.

Ensure adequate rest and recovery time between training sessions and a regular good night's sleep. A daily log of training including how each session went can pinpoint if unusual tiredness is being experienced.

Possible Causes of Gastro-intestinal Problems

Cause	Resulting problem
Using concentrated drinks	Diarrhoea and stomach cramps
High fibre pre-exercise meal	Bloating, cramp and diarrhoea
High fat/high protein pre-exercise meal	Nausea and vomiting
Dehydration	General digestive problems
Reduced blood flow to intestine	Cramping and diarrhoea persisting after exercise
Impact (jarring stomach contents and speeding their journey down)	Diarrhoea and cramping

Keep well hydrated and eat well, including plenty of fresh fruit and vegetables and lots of carbohydrates.

THE UNDERPERFORMING ATHLETE

Hard training and progressive overload leads to improved performance in the majority of athletes but for a small number this is not true and performance can even get worse. In the past it has been variously called over-training syndrome, burnout, chronic fatigue or staleness but more recently these have been replaced by the more accurate term Unexplained Underperformance Syndrome (UPS).

UPS is described as a persistent unexplained performance deficit (recognized and agreed by coach and athlete) despite two weeks of relative rest. A variety of symptoms may be present which will vary from one athlete to another, the key one being fatigue and an unexpected sense of effort during training. Others include:

- history of heavy training and competition;
- frequent minor infections;
- unexplained or unusually heavy, stiff and/or sore muscles;
- mood disturbance;
- change in expected sleep quality;
- loss of energy;
- loss of competitive drive;
- loss of libido; and
- loss of appetite.

Diet can play an important role in helping to prevent underperformance. Indeed suboptimal diets are frequently identified in those who show signs and symptoms of underperformance. For example, re-fuelling after

> **Examples of Refuelling Snacks for a 80kg Athlete**
>
> Aim for 1g carbohydrate per kg body weight, in other words approximately 80g in this example.
>
> - 500ml Lucozade Sport (32g carbohydrate), one large banana (25g carbohydrate) and one Nutrigrain bar (26g carbohydrate).
> - 500ml Isostar (38g carbohydrate) and three raisin and lemon pancakes (50g carbohydrate).
> - 500ml Gatorade (30g carbohydrate) and one 55g pack of Skittles (50g carbohydrate).
> - 500ml Lucozade Sport (32g carbohydrate), one 50g pack of Pretzels (38g carbohydrate) and one Go Ahead caramel crisp (16g carbohydrate).
> - 500ml Isostar (38g carbohydrate) and one 65g Mars bar (45g carbohydrate).
> - 500ml Gatorade (30g carbohydrate), one bagel (45g carbohydrate) and one teaspoon of honey (5g carbohydrate).

training sessions may not be effective. Many athletes achieve a reasonable intake of carbohydrate at meal times but what invariably lets them down, for a variety of reasons, is the immediate refuelling after training.

It is a useful to work out five or six different practical refuelling snacks that meet the carbohydrate refuelling requirement of 1g carbohydrate per kg body weight and which can be taken to the training venue. Using nutritional information on packaging this is not difficult, particularly if the bulk of the carbohydrate comes from a sports drink which is already being drunk for rehydration purposes.

ADEQUATE INTAKES OF IRON AND ANTI-OXIDANT NUTRIENTS

Iron deficiency, a common nutritional deficiency in the UK, has been associated with adverse effects on work capacity, reduced physical performance and reduced resistance to infection. Attention should therefore be paid to dietary iron intakes and the practical ways of increasing iron intakes.

Strenuous exercise certainly increases the production of free radicals either during exercise or the recovery period. Athletes undertaking a strenuous training programme may benefit in the long term by being able to sustain that training load if they pay particular attention to their intake of antioxidant nutrients. The best advice is generally to ensure a regular intake of fruit and vegetables although, failing this, a regular supplement of antioxidant nutrients may be useful.

GLUTAMINE SUPPLEMENTATION

There are many benefits of moderate regular exercise including protection against infection. On the other hand, hard intense exercise seems to increase the risk of infection. There are several factors that could be responsible, one of which may be the low level of the non-essential amino acid glutamine which is found after hard training. Glutamine is involved in some of the functions of the immune system. Low levels of glutamine have been found in chronically fatigued and under-performing athletes. The limited amount of research on glutamine supplementation does not suggest any clear-cut advice about supplementation. The positive effect of supplementation on resistance to infection has not always been present and more research is needed before advice about the use of glutamine supplements can be given.

CHAPTER 13

The Travelling Athlete

Travelling and staying away from home, whether it is abroad or just somewhere in the same country can present athletes with potential problems that can affect performance in both training and competition situations. Sporting activity holidays such as skiing, mountaineering or trekking can also be ruined by not taking time to plan and prepare for the holiday properly before leaving home.

Most people in the UK live at or close to sea level, enjoy a temperate climate, eat foods that are familiar and tend to keep to a daily or weekly routine. Travelling to a foreign country, there may be a need to acclimatize to a new climate (hotter, more humid or colder) or higher altitude, food may be unfamiliar, drinking water may not be safe and most certainly the normal routine will be upset. There may be a need to overcome jet lag and other consequences of travelling. There are two main areas to consider when planning a diet strategy for a trip: the requirements when travelling and the requirements when at the final destination.

AIR TRAVEL

The air in the cabin is usually pressurised to 6,000 feet, not ground level. The air is therefore thinner and very dry (low humidity) so there is a real danger of becoming dehydrated. Arriving after a lengthy plane journey with a thumping headache is a common occurrence.

Accommodation on board a plane is invariably cramped so there is a risk of stiffness and muscle cramps. Deep vein thrombosis can occur, particularly after a long-haul flight.

Careful choice of drinks during the flight can help prevent dehydration occurring. Alcohol should be avoided at the airport and during the flight as this will increase the risk of becoming dehydrated both during the flight and afterwards. Drinking too much (in other words more than usual) tea, coffee and cola can also lead to dehydration. Caffeine, present in all these drinks, is a diuretic which increases urine output. Better choices are fruit juice, squash and mineral water (still rather than sparkling). It is also a good idea to carry at least one litre of water in hand luggage. Walking around, stretching and even doing some exercises while sitting can help to cut down stiffness and cramping.

The length of journey will determine how many meals are served during the flight. For some athletes, airline portion sizes can be too small so a selection of suitable snacks such as fresh and dried fruit, cereal bars and sandwiches can be packed in hand luggage and used to supplement meals. Some countries do not allow certain food items to be brought in (for example passengers are not allowed to take fresh fruit and vegetables into Australia) so what is not eaten in flight will have to be thrown away. Most airlines can cater for special needs with sufficient notice (in the case of British Airways, only twenty-four hours) and can provide vegetarian meals, low fat meals, kosher meals and so on.

Jet Lag

In normal circumstances the body clock adjusts to the solar day by the rhythmic routine of dark and light and the daily routine of social factors, activities and meals. As a result the body is 'primed' during the day and partially 'shut down' at night. Travelling and crossing time zones disturbs the body clock causing a mismatch between it (still running on departure time) and the new environment with its new time cues. This is jet lag, the symptoms of which are daytime fatigue, inability to sleep at night, difficulty in concentrating, headache, loss of appetite and irregularities in bowel movements. These symptoms are much worse after a flight Eastwards rather than Westwards. The severity is directly related to the number of time zones crossed. It is not due to the stress of the flight or the 'culture shock' on arrival in a foreign country. Jet lag is not experienced after North/South flights. To adjust fully, most people need to allow up to one day for each time zone crossed.

Use of Melatonin to Overcome Jet Lag

Prior to the Sydney Games, the British Olympic Association Medical Committee produced a statement on the use of melatonin. They advise 'great caution in the use of drugs such as hypnotics (sleeping pills) or melatonin to overcome jet lag. Melatonin is not licensed or available in the United Kingdom and sleeping pills are only available on prescription. These drugs have unpredictable effects, including prolonged drowsiness in some individuals and they may even slow adjustment to new time zones. Only consider using sleeping pills or melatonin if you have used them before

---

Coping With Jet Lag

- The new local hours should be adopted as soon as possible. Watches should be set to destination time immediately on take-off and the temptation to keep converting back to home time should be resisted.
- Daytime naps lasting more than an hour during the first few days should be avoided.
- Local sleeping and waking patterns should be adopted as soon as possible.
- On arrival, meals should be taken at the correct time for the new time zone.
- Large meals and caffeine-containing drinks should be avoided late at night as this may make sleep difficult.
- Alcohol may initially encourage sleep but its diuretic properties may well result in the need to pass urine during the night followed by an inability to get back to sleep again.

---

and know the effect on you. It is essential that your team doctor and other sports science and medical support staff are closely involved with your strategy to overcome jet lag as quickly as possible.'

ROAD AND RAIL TRAVEL

There may be no shortage of eating places on the road but many athletes will find it easier to keep to their diet if they take their own food. Suitable foods include sandwiches with low fat fillings (tuna, chicken, low fat soft cheese, bananas and peanut butter with jam), fruit (fresh and dried), currant buns, scones and cereal bars. Bottled water and fruit juice are good choices of drinks. Buying food from shops on the way is another option but this can become time-consuming and also frustrating if basic items such as knives and spoons have not been packed.

143

Suitable Fluids and Food for Travelling

Fluids
Water
Fruit juice
Ready-to-drink squash
Sports drinks

Food
Fresh fruit
Dried fruit
Dried fruit and nuts
Cereal and breakfast bars
Breakfast cereal (eaten by the handful)
Sandwiches, rolls, bagels
Breadsticks, pretzels, crackers
Fig rolls, ginger biscuits (particularly useful
   for alleviating travel sickness)
Malt loaf, pancakes, scones, Chelsea buns
   etc

Avoiding Stomach Upsets

- If the local water supply is unsafe, bottled, boiled or sterilized water should be the choice, including water used for cleaning teeth. Even when tap water is safe, the variation in bacteria may cause a gastro intestinal upset.
- Adding ice to drinks is the same as adding tap water and should be avoided.
- Care must be taken to avoid swallowing water during swimming or showering.
- Fruits that can be peeled such as bananas, oranges and grapefruit are safest.
- Avoid salad unless washed in clean water. (How do you know it is clean? Be guided by the country and the establishment you are eating in.)
- Avoid foods made from unpasteurized milk (such as local cream, yoghurt and ice cream).
- Properly cooked food is less risky than raw food. Undercooked meat should always be avoided. Reheated food should also be avoided.
- Eat out only in establishments that are well known or recommended by reliable people (hotel managers, coaches or people who have been to the area before). Food sold on streets, from stalls or in open markets should be avoided.
- It is wise to avoid shellfish, particularly in the Mediterranean or Tropics as the fish may be harvested from contaminated water.
- Observe the normal rules of personal hygiene.

Athletes should have fewer dietary problems when travelling by train, certainly in the UK, although foreign trains may serve unfamiliar and unsuitable food (often at extortionate prices). Again, if in doubt home-made packed meals may be the best solution. Care should be taken to store food carefully to avoid the risk of food poisoning.

Long hours spent travelling by any method can upset the digestive system, in particular leading to constipation. This can be minimized by eating lots of fruit and fibre-rich foods and drinking plenty of water. Energy requirements will be lower than when training so less food will be needed. However when travelling it is easy to either under-eat (not feeling hungry) or over-eat (less active and bored).

FINAL DESTINATION

The final destination will vary considerably, from an Olympic Village to a hall of residence, from a hotel to a hostel, and so will the food provision. Athletes may find it difficult to keep to their prescribed diet and to eat only foods that are preferred or familiar. The possible consequences of an upset to normal eating habits include weight fluctuations, constipation, gastro-intestinal upsets, thirst, irritability, anxiety or fatigue. None of these will help an athlete to produce a personal best performance or maximize the opportunity of a warm-weather training camp. Equally, they could take away the enjoyment of an activity holiday.

To avoid running into dietary problems, athletes need to make some careful plans in advance. Suitable nutritious snacks brought from home can always top-up food intakes so that athletes do not go hungry. If it is possible, meals should be arranged in advance. For instance, if a team or squad is to stay in hotel accommodation, it will help to let the hotel know in advance that plenty of pasta dishes, vegetarian food or extra portions might be needed. As athletes travel to different venues it is a very worthwhile exercise to keep a diary for future reference, noting foods that could have been taken from home, good restaurants and shops that sold familiar foods.

EATING OUT

Athletes who eat out in restaurants, hotels or fast food outlets will benefit from knowing which are the wiser choices on the menu, particularly if they eat out often.

Fast Food Retailer. The best choice is a basic beefburger with no trimmings and an extra bun (it is okay and possible to ask for this) and a milk shake. Adding cheese adds extra fat. Chicken burgers are often coated with mayonnaise, deep fried and served with more mayonnaise; in other words, they are not as healthy as they might sound. French fries (thin chips) absorb more fat in cooking than thick ones.

Chinese Restaurant. Chinese cooking uses a lot of vegetables and not much fat (apart from the obvious deep-fried items such as sweet and sour pork, which should be avoided). Most menus give descriptions of the ingredients in a dish and how it is cooked, but if in doubt ask the waiter. Avoid prawn crackers. Soups and crispy duck are better choices than spare ribs or spring rolls. Choose stir-fries and steamed food for main dishes. Choose plain boiled rice or noodles. Drink plenty of water or tea (Chinese meals can be high in salt). If over-eating is a potential problem, try using chopsticks in order to slow down.

French or Italian Restaurant. Start with bread and breadsticks, minestrone soup but avoid garlic bread and whitebait. Avoid creamy sauces and choose vegetable based sauces if possible. Choose meat, fish or poultry that has been grilled, steamed, poached, baked, casseroled or roasted rather than fried, battered, creamed, buttered, sautéed or *au gratin*. Choose boiled or mashed potatoes, pasta or rice. Avoid vegetables that are fried, roasted or tossed in butter or ask for vegetables to be served plain.

Greek Restaurant. Greek meals are built around salad vegetables, bread, pasta and rice but can contain large amounts of olive oil. Tzatziki and pitta bread is a good choice for starters. Salads can be served without dressings and feta cheese is a lower fat variety. Greek menus usually contain a range of grilled meats and fish. Greek yoghurt and fruit is a good way to finish the meal.

Indian Restaurant. Indian menus usually explain what each dish contains and some times how it is cooked. Samosas, crispy rolls and other fried starters should be avoided. Tandoori dishes and kebabs will not come swimming in ghee or oil. Other good choices are biryanis and sauces such as dhansak, rogan josh and jalfrezi. Kormas, pasandas and

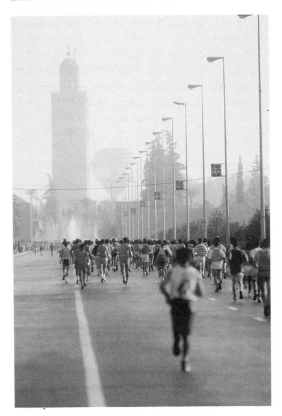

Runners make their way back to Marrakesh in the Marrakesh Marathon, Morocco.

masalas have creamy sauces and are not the best choices on the menu. Plain rice, plain naan and chapattis are wise choices.

Pizza Restaurant. Select toppings that do not include salami, pepperoni and extra cheese to keep the fat content down. Good toppings include tomatoes, mushrooms, seafood, peppers and sweetcorn, ham and pineapple. Deep pan pizzas are higher in carbohydrate than thin crust pizzas. Pasta with tomato sauce is available in many pizza restaurants and this is always a safe choice.

EXTREME CONDITIONS

Athletes and active holidaymakers will often find themselves in extreme conditions of heat, cold or altitude. Certain dietary precautions can be taken to help maintain performance and health in such conditions.

Hot Climates

It can be helpful to keep a diary of fluid intake and urine habits (frequency, approximate volume and colour) for a few days before leaving home to provide baseline information. Training and competing in a hot and/or humid environment will lead to a much greater risk of dehydration. A change in habits from the norm, such as urinating less often, passing a smaller volume of urine or urine of a darker colour than normal can all indicate progressive dehydration. A high fluid intake must be maintained throughout the travel time. On leaving the plane, carry some drinks as hand luggage in case there are delays in Immigration and Customs.

On arrival in a hot/humid environment, athletes will lose a lot of sweat and need to increase their fluid intake accordingly if they are not to become dehydrated. Most people are dehydrated for the first day or two after arrival until they have adjusted their fluid intake. Dehydration will show in the changes in urination already mentioned, in possible weight loss, in feelings of tiredness and lethargy and poor performance in training and competition. Further dehydration will increase the risk of heat illness.

Regular weighing each morning and, if possible, before and after training sessions should be undertaken. Daily weighing keeps an overall regular check and weighing at training shows how much should be drunk during the training session to keep dehydration to a minimum.

Keeping Up Fluids

- Athletes must work at their fluid intake since nobody automatically drinks enough to prevent dehydration. Ideally carry a drink bottle all the time and take regular gulps.
- Water or other suitable drinks should be drunk with all meals and if possible at the end of the meal as well. Extra salting at meals may be needed in the first days of acclimatization, particularly if sweat losses are high.
- A variety of drinks, such as water, sports drinks, soft drinks, juices and tea and coffee can be drunk. Regular tea and coffee drinkers should not drink more of these than normal.
- Keep a water bottle by the bed.
- Sports drinks are ideal for use immediately before, during and after training or competition. However these drinks do have an energy value and if drunk exclusively they could encourage unwanted weight gain.

Cold Climates

Adequate stores of carbohydrate are not only important to provide fuel for the exercising muscles, they may help to maintain core body temperature, particularly in leaner athletes. This is because carbohydrate is the major fuel source for shivering, an involuntary contraction of muscle that occurs in response to a fall in body temperature. It is sensible for anybody exercising in the cold to plan a carbohydrate snack every two hours.

Alcohol dilates the blood vessels, which will lead to an increase in the rate of heat loss. It should therefore be avoided until some time after exercise finishes and full hydration has been established. It is also important to remember the other consequences of alcohol intake and its effect on exercise and recovery (*see* Chapter 4).

Fluid intakes to replace sweat losses will be less of a priority but the carbohydrate content of any drink used around exercise should not be more than 12 per cent carbohydrate as this can lead to gastro-intestinal problems.

ALTITUDE

At altitude the barometric pressure is lower and air becomes less dense as a result. The amount of oxygen in a given volume of air is less than at sea level. This has little effect on someone resting but does affect those who are exercising. This is more noticeable above altitudes of 2,000m (approximately 6,000 feet) but may be noticed at lower altitudes. The effects are more obvious in endurance sports than in power sports. Initially athletes experience tiredness during exercise, headaches, nausea and difficulty in sleeping. These symptoms disappear as athletes acclimatize to the higher altitude. Requirements for some nutrients are changed as a result of altitude.

Carbohydrate Intake

Exercise at altitude uses more muscle glycogen for the same activity than would be used at sea level so special attention must be paid to carbohydrate intake. Unfortunately, food intake may be reduced by 10 to 15 per cent in the initial period at altitude, partly because of loss of appetite. It is therefore important to ensure a good intake of carbohydrate in the days leading up to departure and during travel and to take supplies of suitable foods that are normally enjoyed.

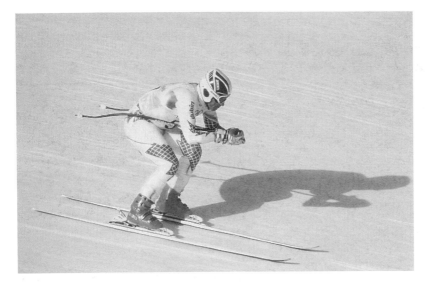

Nils Lindberg of Chile competing in the Men's Downhill in the 1998 Winter Olympics at Nagano.

Fluid Intake

The low humidity of the atmosphere means that the air is drier and so evaporative losses are greater. Hyperventilation leads to more fluid loss in breathing but because the sweat loss from the skin is faster than at sea level athletes may actually think they are sweating less than usual. If they are less aware of sweat loss they are probably less likely to think about fluid intake, let alone drink more than usual. Dehydration has a detrimental effect on performance but it is also a health risk. Sufficient, palatable fluids of the correct composition must always be to hand. Again it is essential that athletes do not arrive at altitude already dehydrated because of travelling.

Intake of Vitamins and Minerals

Athletes with low iron stores may have problems when red blood cell production is stimulated at altitude (a key reason for altitude training). Athletes, particularly vegetarian female athletes should pay attention to their intake of iron-rich foods in the weeks prior to going to altitude as well as at altitude.

Useful Foods to Keep in Stock

STORE CUPBOARD ITEMS

Cereal-Based Foods

Breakfast cereals: great snack foods, not just for eating at breakfast time. Can be eaten by the handful without milk.

Pasta: all shapes and sizes, very quick to cook and serve with sauces. Can also be combined with many other store-cupboard ingredients to make salads.

Noodles.

Rice: takes a bit longer to cook than pasta but the same applies. Use with sauces, in risottos and salad. Canned rice is quicker but more expensive.

Savoury rice: a quick way to make risotto.

Instant mashed potatoes: more expensive than buying potatoes but very convenient.

Grains: couscous, bulgar wheat, polenta.

Oat cakes, crispbreads and digestive biscuits: for snacks with cheese, honey, jam or Marmite.

Cereal bars: useful snack foods but some have high fat contents.

Pizza base: this is a good standby. Add toppings of choice.

Bread sticks, crispbreads, water biscuits, Matzos and so on.

Fruit and Vegetables

Canned tomatoes (chopped and passata, with or without herbs): good for sauces and pizza toppings.

Tomato puree: for added flavour.

Canned beans: not only baked beans in tomato sauce but also red kidney beans, butter beans, chilli beans, borlotti beans, cannellini beans and chickpeas. They are more expensive than dried beans but are ready to be added to sauces, salads, soups or mixed with vegetables to fill pitta pockets at a moment's notice.

Canned sweetcorn: a versatile vegetable which can be added to baked beans, mixed into a salad or just warmed through and served as a side vegetable.

Canned fruit: a good standby for when fresh fruit runs out. Canned pineapple mixed with low fat soft cheese makes a healthy filling for jacket potatoes. Canned blackcurrants blended in a food processor with thick custard makes a quick 'fool'.

Dried fruit: the semi-dried varieties of apricots and prunes together with dried figs, raisins and sultanas make useful snacks and end of meal top-ups. Add to breakfast cereals and sandwich fillings.

Lemon juice: for flavouring and added vitamin C.

Meat and Alternatives
Canned meat: corned beef and ham are good standbys for sandwich fillings and to add to omelettes. Visible fat should be trimmed away.

Canned fish: tuna (preferably in brine or spring water, or with the oil drained off), sardines, salmon, mackerel and pilchards. These are all useful for sauces, salads, on toast, in pitta bread pockets or as fillings for jacket potatoes.

Dairy Produce
UHT semi-skimmed or skimmed milk in cartons are a useful standby if fresh milk runs out. Dried skimmed or semi-skimmed milk is another useful standby.

Drinks
Long-life cartons of fruit juice.

Regular or low calorie squash or high juice drinks.

Regular or low calorie fizzy drinks.

Miscellaneous
Crunchy or smooth peanut butter, Marmite, honey, jam, marmalade and chocolate spread: these are good as sandwich fillings or toast toppings.

Pasta and stir-fry sauces: quicker than making from store-cupboard ingredients.

Nuts, fruit and nuts, seeds: for snacks, adding to salads and tossing into sauces for pasta and rice.

Canned soups: add pasta, rice or beans to push up the carbohydrate content.

Canned condensed soups: these can double as sauces.

Canned low fat milk puddings and canned, cartons or pots of custard: quick, healthy filling puddings.

Worcestershire sauce: to add flavour.

Flour.

Mustard, horseradish sauce, soy sauce, vinegar.

Mint sauce.

Chilli powder.

Curry powder.

Dried herbs and spices: mixed herbs is an all-purpose standby. It is surprising how a change of herb or spice can make the same meal taste quite different.

FRIDGE ITEMS

Cereal-Based Foods
Bread: this keeps better in the fridge, especially during warm weather.

Fresh pasta: just cook and top with a little Parmesan cheese.

Meat and Alternatives
Wafer thin ham and smoked turkey: good for sandwich fillings or add to sauces.

Low fat liver pâté: for sandwich fillings or toast toppings.

Eggs: for example, scrambled egg on toast or omelettes.

Quorn and tofu: easy and quick to cook. Try stir-frys and meat-free Bolognese.

Dairy Produce
Skimmed or semi-skimmed milk: for adding to breakfast cereal, making milkshakes and so on.

Yoghurts: low fat fruit yoghurt for snacks and puddings, low fat natural yoghurt for toppings and sauces. Greek yoghurt (0 per cent fat) makes an ideal substitute for creamy sauces (note that this should be warmed through and not allowed to boil).

Parmesan cheese: useful for toppings on lots of dishes. It keeps for a long time and only a little is needed for flavour so the fat content is kept down

Low fat soft cheese and Quark: plain or flavoured for sandwich fillings, spreading on pitta bread or melting down for sauces.

Cheese: Edam, low fat hard cheese, cottage cheese, cheese slices and so on.

Low fat fromage frais: an alternative to natural yoghurt.

Spreads
Low fat spread, polyunsaturated margarine or butter.

FREEZER ITEMS

Cereal-Based Foods
Bread: (slices can be toasted from frozen), rolls, baps and muffins.

Pitta bread: can be defrosted and heated up in the toaster or under the grill in moments.

Fruit buns, teacakes and scones. Ideal for the kit bag as they thaw out during the training session.

Meat and Alternatives
Lean mince: for meat sauces and cottage/shepherd's pie. Freeze in meal-sized portions.

Lean cubed meat: for kebabs. Freeze in meal-sized portions.

Chicken or turkey fillets: for grilling, kebabs or cooking in a sauce.

Chicken drumsticks.

Chicken nuggets.

Fish fingers and fish cakes.

Fish steaks.

Fruit and Vegetables
All frozen vegetables: nutritionally frozen vegetables are just as good as fresh if they are cooked properly.

Oven chips (5 per cent sunflower oil): these can be quickly grilled from frozen. Lower in fat than traditional chips.

Frozen fruits.

Dairy Produce
Grated cheese.

Drinks
Concentrated fruit juice.

Sorbet.

Ice cream (non-dairy as this is lower in fat).

APPENDIX II
Mealtime Suggestions

BREAKFAST

Breakfast cereals with milk and dried or sliced fresh fruit on top, especially bananas.

Muesli with fresh fruit and low fat natural yoghurt.

Porridge cooked with raisins and eaten with sugar, Golden syrup or maple syrup and milk.

Chopped fruit (fresh and dried) with low fat natural yoghurt.

Toast, bread or muffins with a little low fat spread and marmalade, honey or jam, Marmite or Vegemite, peanut butter or chocolate spread (no need for low fat spread as well), low fat cheese (especially low fat soft cheese) and tomatoes.

Banana milkshake (banana, milk and honey).

Warm roll or toasted muffin with sliced banana and honey.

Yoghurt drink.

COOKED BREAKFAST

Baked beans on toast or pitta bread.

Crispy grilled bacon sandwich.

Poached egg with bread or toast.

Boiled egg with bread or toast.

Fish fingers and grilled tomatoes and toast.

Grilled tomatoes, lean grilled bacon, mushrooms and toast.

Omelettes stuffed with baked beans, mushrooms or tomatoes.

Potato cakes with tomatoes and mushrooms.

Kedgeree (with lots of rice and less of the other ingredients).

Pancakes with maple syrup.

PACKED MEAL

Sandwiches are traditional and convenient items to include in a packed meal but they can become boring if the same fillings and bread are used every day. Ring the changes by using wholemeal, granary, soft grain or white bread. Try different shaped breads such as French sticks or baguettes, crusty rolls or soft baps, bagels or pitta bread. The spread acts as a barrier to stop the bread going soggy, but only a thin layer of low fat spread is needed. Alternatively, peanut butter or low fat soft cheese can be used.

There are endless variations on possible sandwich fillings. Here are just a few ideas:

- Ham and tomato slices.
- Low fat liver pâté and watercress.
- Cold chicken and pineapple chunks bound

together with low calorie salad dressing or yoghurt.

- Smoked turkey or chicken slices with cranberry sauce.
- Grilled lean bacon with tomatoes and lettuce.
- Mashed sardines with tomato purée.
- Tuna with lemon juice.
- Grated cheese with Marmite.
- Low fat soft cheese or curd cheese with pickle.
- Edam cheese with apple slices.
- Chopped hard-boiled egg with lean ham.
- Chopped hard-boiled egg with low calorie salad dressing and mustard and cress.
- Peanut butter and mashed banana.
- Peanut butter and honey.
- Peanut butter and jam (known as PJs in the USA!).
- Mashed banana.

Where possible, some vegetables should be included in the packed meal, whether in the sandwich or as a separate item. Freshly prepared salads provide a nice, crunchy texture. All types of raw, chopped vegetables can be used and also of course cooked pasta, rice, potatoes or beans.

Other items that can be included are:

- Fresh fruit (all sorts).
- Dried fruit or fruit and nuts.
- Cereal bars such as Nutrigrains, Squares, Jordans.
- Fruit cake, parkin, gingerbread, fruit loaf, banana bread, and so on.
- Pancakes, for example lemon and raisin.
- Scones or semi-sweet biscuits such as digestives.
- Low fat yoghurt or Mullerice.
- Low fat crisps.
- Fun size chocolate bar such as a Crunchie or Mars bar.

The packed meal must include fluids: fruit juice, dilute squash (traditional or low calorie), fizzy canned drink (traditional or low calorie), water or a hot drink.

MAIN MEAL

Shepherd's pie or cottage pie made with extra lean mince, peas and carrots.

Pasta with tomato sauce and tuna.

Chicken stir-fry with vegetables and rice or noodles.

Grilled lean meat with mashed or boiled potatoes and vegetables.

Roast chicken with jacket potato and vegetables.

Grilled fish fingers with mashed potatoes and vegetables.

Chicken, vegetable or lentil curry with rice.

Baked fish (white fish, tomatoes, onions, mushrooms) with jacket potatoes and vegetables.

Pasta with a lean Bolognese sauce.

Rice with lean chilli con carne.

Rice with red kidney bean and vegetable sauce.

Macaroni cheese, made with low fat milk and cheese.

Chicken casserole with jacket potatoes and vegetables.

Deep pan pizza, thick crust with lean ham and pineapple.

Risotto with tuna, lean ham or chicken.

PUDDING

Fruit crumble with custard.

Milk puddings such as rice pudding and semolina with jam or dried fruit.

Pancakes with maple or Golden syrup.

Baked apples with dried fruit and custard.

Instant whips made with low fat milk.

Sponge and custard.

Banana and custard.

Fruit in jelly with custard.

Yoghurts, *fromage frais*, Mullerice.

Dietitians in Sport and Exercise Nutrition (DISEN)

Dietitians in Sport and Exercise Nutrition (DISEN) is the name of the British Dietetic Association's Sports Nutrition Interest Group which started in 1999. The British Dietetic Association (BDA) was formed in 1936 and incorporated in 1947. It is the professional Association for qualified Dietetians in the United Kingdom, and a condition of full membership is the holding of a recognised dietetic qualification

Members of DISEN are all professionally qualified Dietitians who are State Registered and who have undertaken further training in the specialist area of sports nutrition. State Registered Dietitians work within the professional statement of conduct as laid down by The Council for Professions Supplementary to Medicine.

DISEN acts as a point of contact for information and support relating to sports nutrition. A range of publications including credit card sized laminated pee charts and A4 laminated pee chart posters and a cookery book *Cook and Train without the Strain, Recipes for Active People* have been developed.

Publication and price lists or more information about the group can be obtained by writing to:

Dietitians in Sport and Exercise Nutrition
PO Box 22360
London
W13 9FL

APPENDIX IV
Useful Addresses

British Dietetic Association
5th Floor, Charles House
148/9 Great Charles Street
Queensway
Birmingham
B3 3HT
www.bda.uk.com

British Nutrition Foundation
High Holborn House
52-54 High Holborn
London
WC1V 6RQ
www.nutrition.org.uk

British Olympic Association
1 Wandsworth Plain
London
SW18 1EH
www.olympics.org. uk

British Paralympic Association
Norwich Union Building
9th Floor
69 Park Lane
Croydon
Surrey
CR9 1BG
www.paralympics.org.uk

Corona Worldwide
c/o Commonwealth Institute
Kensington High Street
London
W8 6NQ
(A registered charity that provides information
on living and working overseas and returning
to Britain.)

Dietitians in Sport and Exercise Nutrition
PO Box 22360
London
W13 9FL

Eating Disorders Association
1st Floor
Wensum House
103 Prince of Wales Road
Norwich
NR1 1DW
www.edauk.com

Food Standards Agency
Room 621
Hannibal House
PO Box 30080
Elephant and Castle
London
SE1 6YA
www.foodstandards.gov.uk

FSA Foodsense booklets can be obtained free
of charge (quoting the PB reference number)
from:

FSA Publications
PO Box 369
Hayes
Middlesex
UB3 1UT
Particularly useful booklets are:
Food Safety (PB 0551)
Understanding food labels (PB 0553)
Healthy eating (PB 0550)

Health Development Agency
Trevelyan House
30 Great Peter Street
London
SW1P 2HW

www.had-online.org.uk
(Note that the Health Education Authority no longer exists)

Health Supplements Information Service
Bury House
126–128 Cromwell Road
London
SW7 4ET
www.hsis.org

Ministry of Agriculture, Fisheries and Food
Food Safety Directorate Helpline
3 Whitehall Place
London
SW1 2HH
0645 335577 MAFF Helpline
www.maff.gov.uk

sports coach UK
114 Cardigan Road
Headingley
Leeds
LS6 3BJ9
www.sportscoachuk.org

The National Sports Medicine Institute of the United Kingdom
32 Devonshire Street
London
W1G 6PX
www.nsmi.org.uk

The Nutrition Society
10 Cambridge Court
210 Shepherds Bush Road
London
W6 7NJ
www.nutsoc.org.uk

Sports Council for Northern Ireland
House of Sport
Upper Malone Road
Belfast
BT9 5LA
www.sportni.org

Sports Council for Wales
Sophia Gardens
Cardiff
CF11 9SW
www.sports-council-wales.co.uk

Sport England
16 Upper Woburn Place
London
WC1H 0QP
www.sportengland.org

Sport Scotland
Caledonia House
South Gyle
Edinburgh
EH12 9DQ
www.sportscotland.org.uk

UK Athletics
Athletics House
10 Harborne Road
Edgbaston
Birmingham
B15 3AA
www.ukathletics.org

UK Sport (and UKSI)
40 Bernard Street
London
WC1N 1ST
www.uksport.gov.uk

The Vegan Society
7 Battle Road
St Leonards-on-Sea
East Sussex
TN37 7AA
www.vegansociety.com

Vegetarian Society
Parkdale
Dunham Road
Altrincham
Cheshire
WA14 4QG
www.vegsoc.org

Index